THE EAR
GATEWAY TO BALANCING THE BODY
A MODERN GUIDE TO EAR ACUPUNCTURE

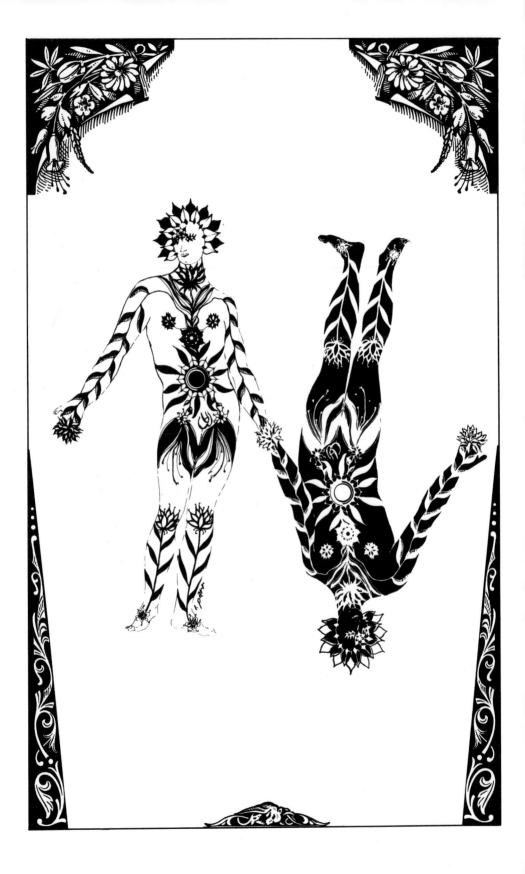

"In the Pure Land there are many lotus blossoms, and each blossom has many precious petals, and each petal shines softly in unspeakable beauty. The radiance of these lotus blossoms brightens the path of Wisdom, and those who listen to the music of the holy teaching are led into perfect peace."

—Gautama Siddartha, the Buddha

THE EAR GATEWAY TO BALANCING THE BODY A MODERN GUIDE TO EAR ACUPUNCTURE

by Mario Wexu

Preface by Dr. Lok Yee-Kung
Illustrations by Ilsa Parr

ASI PUBLISHERS, Inc.
127 Madison Avenue
New York, New York 10016

First Edition

THIRD PRINTING 1982

Printed in U.S.A. by
Noble Offset Printers, Inc.
New York, N.Y. 10003

3   4   5   6   7   8   9   10

Library of Congress Cataloging in Publication Data

Wexu, Mario, 1945-
    The ear, gateway to balancing the body.

    Bibliography: p.
    1. Acupuncture. 2. Ear. I. Title.
RM184.W46   615'.892   75-20107
ISBN 0-88231-022-4

To Uma Somerfield, with love and affection.

To my acupuncture teachers, my father, Dr. Oscar Wexu, Dr. Lok Yee-kung and Dr. King-Ying.

ACKNOWLEDGEMENTS

It is with the deepest respect and gratitude that I offer acknowledgements to those people who have been most instrumental in giving me the background required to become an acupuncturist.

First of all I must thank my father, Dr. Oscar Wexu, president of the Quebec Association of Acupuncture, without whose instruction I should never have entered this vast study. Next, I must thank Dr. Lok Yee-Kung of Las Vegas, Nevada, who gave me further instruction at the time he was still in Hong Kong and whom I continue to visit regularly.

I offer all due respect to the late Dr. King-Ying whose abundant knowledge was shared with me freely, and at a time when she was still ailing. Her faith in my capacity to learn acupuncture and to help spread it throughout America has never left me.

Several other people have been instrumental in my formation as an acupuncturist. Dr. Jean Schatz, vice-president of the International Society of Acupuncture, did much in the way of explaining to me many of the nuances which have not been understood yet by any Western school. I owe much to Eugene Tong, a Chinese artist and scholar, who generously instructed me in the Chinese way of thinking through the Chinese classics and who helped me to translate many old Chinese acupuncture textbooks.

Last of all, but not least, I must thank Barbara Somerfield and Henry Weingarten of ASI Publishers, Inc., New York. It was their idea to have me write this book and without their aid and encouragement I should never have completed this task.

TABLE OF CONTENTS

LIST OF ILLUSTRATIONS

PREFACE

Auricle (ear) acupuncture is a therapy in which needles are inserted into certain points on the human ear for the purpose of treating disease. Its use has been recorded in classical Chinese medical books, dating back to the *Nei Ching*.

It was in 1957, however, that it experienced a revival. Additional ear acu-points were discovered and were experimented in the various hospitals of Mainland China. The outstanding results it brought about in halting and treating inflammation quickly led to its acceptance by acupuncturists the world over.

In our practice, we have ample proof that the rate of success depends entirely on the correct selection of ear acu-points, whether we are speaking of local pain, acute or chronic inflammatory conditions. The proper technique must also be carefully selected. For example, in treating pharyngitis, laryngitis, or tonsilitis where dyspnea are absent, certain bleeding techniques are applied to certain points on the scaphoid fossa. In these type of inflammatory conditions, we will be surprised to find that the pain and swelling have subsided almost immediately after the treatment. Only three-four days of treatment are generally required to bring about a recovery from these diseases.

In the above mentioned cases, the most appropriate points are:

1) A point halfway between the Elbow point and the Appendix[2] point.

2) The Shoulder point.

3) A point 2 fen (1 fen = approx. 2mm.) beneath the Appendix[3] point.

4) The Lung point in the cavum conchae.

The type of needle used for bleeding techniques is usually a special triangular-tipped needle. However, in the absence of such a needle, one may use a needle of a larger gauge than the normal for that purpose. Sterilization is a most important rule to observe.

In the case of hemophiliac patients, we do not practice bleeding. The needles are merely left in place in the above points for a period of 15-30 minutes. In any case which is extremely severe, the patient can be treated several times in one day.

In 1973, I was invited by the Nevada Legislature to give a three week demonstration of traditional Chinese medical techniques, especially by means of acupuncture. The results that I obtained during this short period of time so impressed the judges that a bill was passed almost immediately to legalize acupuncture as a healing technique which should be practiced only by a competent acupuncturist.

Shortly afterwards, I decided to establish myself in the State of Nevada. Patients come from all over the United States and from every walk of life to my clinic in Las Vegas. I shall procede to describe some of the outstanding results which I obtained with ear acupuncture.

Case 1: Statistically, I have found crippling arthritis to be the number one plague which comes to me for acupuncture. One such case was that of a Texas housewife who was confined to a wheelchair due to this affliction. She had been in that state for the last eight years. Her pain had exhausted her and pain-killers had little effect in relieving her of her suffering. After a detailed diagnosis I decided it best to needle her at the following points:

1) A point at the center of the triangular fossa.

2) A point below the first cymba conchae point* and medial to the Drunk point.

3) A point below the second cavum conchae point, level with the Lung point.

4) Ehr Men, SC (TB)-21.

5) A point on the posterior auricle at the Upper Back level and corresponding with the Headache point.

Although it may sound surprising to the novice, 15 minutes after the treatment, she no longer felt the pain at the knees and could even bend them slightly. After only two such treatments she could walk very slowly, with a cane. Needless to say, she discarded her wheelchair completely. After a series of twelve treatments most of the swelling had subsided and she was able to walk slowly and without assistance.

Case 2: A housewife suffering from pancreatitis came to me to be treated. She felt a constant pain in the epigastric region, especially on the left side. Whenever she had an attack, this pain radiated to the back and to the left shoulder, causing nausea and vomiting. She had to lean forward to relieve the pain. She also lost her appetite, suffered from constipation and insomnia. She had been to a number of doctors, none of which even succeeeded in relieving the acute pain. She had become immune to tranquilizers and came to me as a last resort. I succeeded with the following points:

1) Lu Hsi, SC (TB)-19, situated behind the auricle.

2) Chi Mei, SC (TB)-18, situated behind the auricle.

3) I Feng, SC (TB)-17, situated behind the auricle.

4) The Pancreatitis point.

5) A point in the center of the triangilar fossa.

6) A point below the 5th point of the cymba conchae, medial to, and 2 fen from the Drunk point.

7) A point under the 6th cavum conchae point, medial to the Lung area.

A total of 14 points were used in both ears and left in place for a period of 15 minutes. She felt her pain reduced after the very first treatment and slept well the rest of the night. After the 3rd treatment, she started to regain her appetite and to feel more energetic. It wasn't long before her general condition had improved to the point that she no longer felt any pain and could drive alone to the clinic.

Case 3: I received the visit of a 62 year old businessman from New York city. He suffered from emotional stress due to overwork which gradually developed into tachycardia over a period of six years. The attacks were accompanied by profuse sweating, trembling, nausea, vomiting, with a pale complexion and a pulse rate of 190 beats per minute.

He had to be rushed to the hospital immediately whenever he had an attack. Although he recovered from these attacks each time, their frequency gradually increased. Upon examining him, I decided to use the following point:

1) Ehr Men, SC (TB)-21.

2) Heart point.

3) Brain point.

4) Sympathetic point.

Only 15 minutes were required for the pulse rate to go down from 190-90 beats per minute. He slept well that night. After the second treatment, his pulse rate returned to normal.

I never saw that patient again, but seven months later I was visited by a friend of his who had come down to Las Vegas on business. I was astonished to learn that my patient had never suffered another attack since these treatments.

Case 4: A forty nine year old man came to me to be treated for sinusitis which was accompanied by headaches, neuralgia, congestion and nasal discharge. I selected the following ear acupoints:

1) Inner Nose

2) Outer Nose

3) Occiput

4) Forehead

5) Adrenal Glands

6) A point at the center of the ear lobe.

After seven consecutive treatments the patient's nasal discharge decreased immensely and the headaches and congestion disappeared.

Case 5: A thirty four year old woman had been suffering from hypoglycemia and neurosis for the past eight years. She shunned the cold, felt numb all over, trembled and was always hungry. These symptoms were further complicated by headaches, dizziness, fatigue, morbid fear and depression. Following diagnosis I gave her five consecutive treatments with the following points:

1) Sympathetic point

2) Kidneys

3) Liver

4) A point at the center of the cavum conchae, near the Heart point.

After these treatments, the chilliness, numbness, trembling, dizziness, fear and depression were greatly reduced. Another five consecutive treatments were administered with the following ear points:

1) Sympathetic point

2) Spleen

3) Kidneys

4) Adrenal Glands

5) A point at the center of the cymba conchae.

Her previous symptoms had greatly improved by now and she felt much less fatigue and depression. Her headaches too had almost disappeared; all that was left was a dull pain, without the gravity she had felt previously. Nevertheless, it was necessary to administer five more treatments with the following points:

1) Stomach

2) Kidneys

3) Spleen

4) Sympathetic point

5) Adrenal Glands

6) Heart point at the center of the cavum conchae.

Thus a total of 15 treatments were necessary to bring this patient back to a state of well-being. Her beautiful complexion and energetic character hardly allowed one to imagine that this was the same woman who had initially come to be treated.

During my 38 years of clinical experience in the field of acupuncture, I have applied every type of acupuncture treatment in existence. Not only have I been called to lecture on ear acupuncture on many occasions, but I have used it effectively in every type of disease, major or minor. Unfortunately, the books that deal with this subject today, and which are available on the market, are far from sufficient in explaining its use.

Dr. Mario Wexu is a young, but experienced acupuncturist. Not only does he possess the necessary scientific and medical background, but he also has a remarkable understanding of Chinese medical principles. It is my belief that this auricle acupuncture book which he has written, will greatly benefit acupuncturists as a guide, manual, and for their research.

Dr. Lok Yee-Kung, D.T.C.M.

Las Vegas, 1975.

---

*Consult chapter on Chinese points, for clarification. 1st, 2nd, 3rd, etc., points referred to in the preface, are those points as they appear in the list of points for each area of the auricle in this book.

SECTION I:

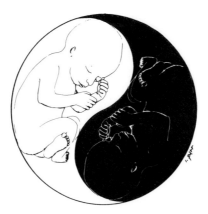

Introduction

CHAPTER 1

THE HISTORY OF EAR ACUPUNCTURE

Ear acupuncture is a form of acupuncture using the ear alone to treat disease. It is also called "auriculotherapy" by those who see it as a distinct form of therapy apart from ordinary acupuncture. It is often stated that the only thing ear acupuncture has in common with ordinary acupuncture is the use of the needle and nothing more. This overlooks the fact that the ancients mentioned the ears for the purpose of diagnosis and the treatment of disease. Moreover, the acupuncturists of Mainland China have proven that links do exist from ancient times, which connect these two branches of acupuncture.

I shall not delve deeply into this argument here, as the purpose of this book is intended to be more of a practical nature, or as a guide, for daily use in your cabinets or clinics. Before I go on to discuss the therapy itself, I shall present some information regarding its use in the past and the related forms of therapy found in various cultures throughout the world.

More than eighty percent of the ear points are fairly recent discoveries, dating back no more than some twenty odd years. We owe a great deal to Dr. Paul Nogier, a French acupuncturist and neurosurgeon who was the first to explore the ear both scientifically and according to Chinese medical principles and who has succeeded in reviving this forgotten branch of Chinese medicine. His discovery of the physiological links of the ear to the human embryo sparked a wave of intensive research in Mainland China, which led to further development in this field.

To date the vast research undertaken in China has led to the discovery of approximately 200 points on the auricle itself, a great number of which vary considerably from Dr. Nogier's locations for them. In this volume I shall present both Dr. Nogier's points and the Chinese points. Our research in this area has confirmed as a fact that both methods are effective and complement one another in treating disease.

The application of ear acupuncture to treat disease has practically no limits. Furthermore, it has the advantage of being a relatively easy to apply method, since no major complications arise from it. It is less time consuming than other methods since the patient usually does not have to undress for treatment, once the diagnosis has been made. Its full effectiveness can be measured in the recently developed form of anesthesia known by the name of acupuncture anesthesia or analgesia. The ear points are considered to be the most effective in eliminating pain during surgery.

EAR ACUPUNCTURE IN ANCIENT CHINA

In ancient China, diagnosis by the auricle was a common practice. Although much of the literature on this subject was lost due to the "great burning of the books", some information does remain. For instance in the *Zen Zhi Zhun Sheng* (Book of Symptoms and their Treatment), it is stated:

A bright and shiny coloration of the helix of the ear is a sign of good vitality. On the contrary, if the helix is extremely dry, death is not far off.

Deafness occurs when there is an excessive combusion of heat in the Shao Yang triple burner meridian, and a plethoral state of energy in the Jue Yin, liver meridian. If the ear is thin and pale, the homolateral kidney is ill.

The *Dhou Ke Shu* (Book of Smallpox) states:

Smallpox is not as serious if the muscles at the back of the auricle are red. The disease only increases in severity once these muscles become purple. A blue-black coloration is particularly difficult to cure.

The *Wang Zhen Zhun Jing* (Classic of Diagnosis by Looking and Observing tells us:

A charcoal, carbonized aspect of the helix of the auricle is indicative of poor assimilation of food and liquids. A bumpy, irregular aspect of the scapha of the auricle indicates an intestinal abcess.

Numerous types of treatment made use of the auricle. For certain diseases, scarification was practiced on ear points. In others, bleeding of ear points and massaging the ears were practiced. One particular technique applied to reanimation consisted of blowing in the patient's ear in a certain way.

The ancients in China had in common with the ancient Arabs, Gypsies, Hindus and Europeans, the practice of needling a point on the lobule of the ear to treat eye troubles such as pinkeye, myopia, and cataract. In the latter cases, gold earings were often prescribed and were deemed to provide a continuous stimulation of the visual centers in the brain. As a matter of fact, many modern European doctors still recommend gold or silver earings to patients suffering from eye deficiencies. Gold is said to have a strengthening, or tonifying effect, while silver is said to have a sedating, or soothing effect.

IN ANCIENT EGYPT

A reknowned Egyptologist, Alexandre Varille, states that in ancient Egypt, women no longer wishing to bear children were needled in a particular spot in the ear. Ancient Egyptian artwork has been found, depicting a queen with a needle in her ear.

IN INDIA

Dr. Chandrashekhar G. Thakkur, world famous authority on Ayurvedic medicine, has stated that in India ear acupuncture was in use several millenia before Christ and is still flourishing today. In the *Suchi Veda*, which is translated as the "Science of Needle Piercing," the various points and techniques of needling the ears are described in great detail. The Indians also have approximately 180 points on the body which they either pierce (acupuncture) or burn (moxibustion) to rid the body of diseases ranging from cough to malaria. These techniques are described in Dr. Thakkur's appendix at the end of the book.

IN ANCIENT GREECE

We know that Hippocrates spent several years studying medicine in Egypt. Whether it is there that he learned of treating diseases by the ear or whether it is an ancient Aryan heritage is thus far a matter of speculation. Nevertheless, four centuries before Christ, which may even be anterior to the Nei Ching (Internal Classic of Chinese Medicine), the first authoritative book dealing with medicine in China, Hippocrates speaks of a treatment to induce sterility in men by making a small incision behind the auricle. This intervention allowed coitus to remain normal but reduced the sperm content in the seminal fluid. This may be the answer to combating the side-effects of the contraceptive pill and quieting female criticism of male chauvinism!

IN SCYTHIA

There may be a relationship between the perversity and brutality of the ancient Scyths and their common sexual impotence which was to them a veritable national plague. Wilhelm Reich should be the first to acknowledge this hypothesis with substantial proof. Whatever the reason, the Scyths apparently remedied this by cutting a small vein behind the ear. It was believed that the seminal fluid had its source in these veins. As in ancient Greece they treated sciatica by burning a point on the anthelix of the auricle.

EUROPE AFTER THE DARK AGES

For the past few centuries, and persisting to this time in France and Italy, Europeans have cauterized a point on the anthelix of the auricle to treat sciatica. The effectiveness of this cure when orthodox methods were not successful led various schools of medicine to look into the matter, resulting in a large number of related articles which have been published in medical journals since the 17th century. In the entire Mediterranean Basin the ear has been used for the treatment of sciatica over the past millenium.

THE ARABS

The Arabs use not only cauterization of the ear to treat sciatica, but also bleeding of the ears in cases of high blood pressure or kidney and back pain. This is still common practice in the small villages of Syria and Lebanon. Although this may have been of Egyptian origin, we are certain that the Arabs had the entire science of acupuncture from the 13th century onward, when the Chinese medical books were translated into Arabic for reference in their medical schools. Avicenna himself was familiar with Chinese pulse techniques, which he used as a kind of lie

detector test. It is remarkable that the Arabs should use the ear
mainly for low back pain and kidney trouble, knowing that the
Chinese consider the ear to be primarily a representative or outer
"flowering" of the kidneys. However, the barbarous bleeding
techniques of the Arabs have nothing to do with modern ear
methods. Certain old Chinese methods may have been quite as
barbarous.

MODERN EAR ACUPUNCTURE

This is a very sophisticated scientific procedure, refined and
perfected through the research of modern scientists such as Dr.
Nogier of France and others in China. As mentioned in the
previous paragraph, modern ear acupuncture has nothing in common with the primitive blood-letting, scarring and burning
techniques used in the past. Definite physiological relationships
have been found connecting certain areas of the auricle to areas of
the body. Needles are inserted into specific points with a diameter
of no more than 1-2 mm. The precise epicenter of these points
solely effects the cure, as does the precise depth.

CHAPTER 2

SYMBOLISM AND REALITY
ATTACHED TO THE EAR

This symbolism is largely of a spiritual and sexual order. It stems deep from the roots of mankind and has accompanied us as though it were part and parcel of our every fibre. Symbolism gave meaning to life. Even though surrounded by magic and mysticism, today it offers the key to a scientific interpretation of reality.

Thus in the Hindu myth of Vaishvarana, the ears represent Cosmic Intelligence and the four directions of space through which penetrates the Holy word or Fact to orientate Man. Great importance is placed upon the spoken word which has the power to stimulate Man in any direction according to how it is used. The ears are the doorway to this powerful vibration of the Soul, which is lodged in the Temples and gathered as an alchemical agent for the purification of the soul.

There is an important relationship here to Chinese medical philosophy, in that the temples are the place of origin of the gall bladder meridian and the final destination of the triple burner or heater meridian, both combining to form the Shao Yang or intermediary meridian of the Yang meridians. The gall bladder represents the Judge of the body, or plumb-line, where every abnormality of the metabolism is reflected, and into which every meridian pours at the end of every cycle of circulation of energy.

7

Any loss of balance of this meridian is reflected by a loss of physical balance, resulting in vertigo, dizziness or loss of perception as to direction in space. (This is not at all contradictory to modern concepts regarding the role the semi-circular canals play in equilibrium.)

In China long ears were analagous to Wisdom and Immortality. The philosopher Lao-Tse was reputed to have 7 inch long ears and was nick-named "long-ears" by his contemporaries. Other famous Chinese Sages bore this trademark. The ears represented spiritual wings. The longer they were, the higher the Spirit could fly. Long ears are represented both in Hindu heroes, Sages and in Egyptian royalty. One of my colleagues sees in them a symptom of sexual impotence. This is largely a matter of speculation.

In some African tribes, the ears represent bestiality and the animal spirit in man. For the Dogons and Bambaras of Mali they have a double sexual function, the auricle representing the penis and the auditory meatus the vagina. Their Goddess Mawu, upon creating woman, was to have placed her sexual organs in the place of her ears. To them the spoken word is as necessary as the seminal fluid in the act of procreation. The word of the male penetrates through the woman's ear and descends to meet the sperm at the matrix, around which they girate in a spiral and impregnate her.

There may be some relation here to the ancient Greek and Scythian practices or treating the ears in sexual difficulties and for the purpose of contraception. Some closer scientific relationship may become apparent in the near future and may lead us to the discovery of a method of male contraception.

Sexual significance was given to the ears in early Christian times as well. A heretic by the name of Elien was condemned before the Council of Nicea for saying that Mary was impregnated by the Word through the ear:

Gaude Virgo mater Christi
Quae per aurum concepisti.

We know that sailors wore an earing in one ear as a symbol of their marriage to the Sea and that certain Sufi mystics did the same as a sign of celibacy. However one regards these myths, in all broadmindedness, we must see in them some truth, especially as regards the power of the spoken word to increase mental and sensual stimulation.

In this sense I believe that not only the ears play an important role, but the eyes and nose as well. The kind of stimulation our sense organs receive largely determine our state of physical and mental well-being. Is it not true that the sense organs, or rather the functions they represent, are the guardians of our soul, giving the body and its systems the word "Go" when they judge it wise?

Let us bear in mind that every part of the body is related and that a malfunction in one part is reflected in another by means of various forms of micro-waves. Effective forms of therapy have been devised using only the nose, eyes, scalp, hair, blood, feet, or hands. (See Diagram 22.)

DIAGRAM 1
Chinese Foetus representation

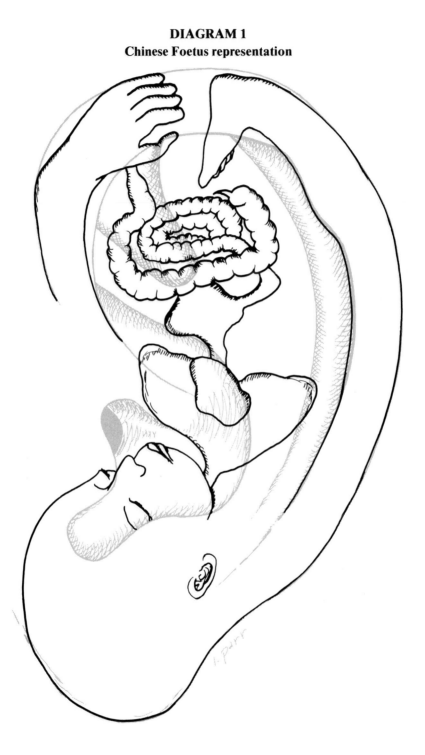

PHYSIOLOGICAL LINKS OF THE EAR
TO THE INTERNAL ORGANS
(OCCIDENTAL AND ORIENTAL)

If one looks closely at the ear, one finds a curious resemblance to the foetus as placed in the womb before coming out into the world, i.e., in an inverted position. The lobule represents the head, concha the internal organs, etc. (As shown in Diagram 1.) Scientific experiments carried out both in Europe and in China have shown that there is in fact a close physiological relationship between specific areas of the ear to specific areas of the body. To date some 200 such loci or points, as they are called, have been found on the ear, and when stimulated, they send a signal to the brain, which in turn sends a signal to the corresponding areas or functions of the body.

On the auricle itself we find an ample supply of nerves and blood vessels, originating from nerves and larger blood vessels in the body. It would appear that the stimulation of the nerve endings on the auricle send a wave along to the main nerve trunks ennervating the corresponding organs which they control. Conversely, a malfunction of an internal organ is represented on the auricle itself in the form of pain in a precise locus, similar to referred pain in other parts of the body, or a Nodule, discoloration, eczema, scar, etc. All these signs serve in making a precise diagnosis from the auricle. We must also take into consideration external factors such as weather and accidents, which modify the appearance of the ear. This will be explained in a later chapter.

It must be pointed out at this moment that we are still uncertain as to the origins of many of the nerve endings on the auricle. To trace each nerve fibre is a tedious task not facilitated by the fact that a good 3-dimensional microscope hasn't been developed yet. Nevertheless enough has been traced to satisfy modern scientific scepticism of its mechanism. In other words the ear serves as a kind of annex-brain adjoined to the main brain, and as a switchboard telling us what is going on within. By making the right connection, we can correct anything that is out of order.

The fact that the ear represents the foetus should not appear strange if one studies Chinese philosophy. In Taoist Yoga, great stress is placed on pre-natal conditions. They signify ideal peace, serenity and harmony, representing the eternal womb of Life or Immortality on a microcosmic scale.

The Chinese Yogi performs a certain form of breathing exercises for the purpose of transforming the rough impure essences of his body into pure alchemical agents, known as the Golden Elexir, or Elexir of Immortality. He names this type of breathing pre-natal breathing, or "breathing as in a womb." Thus the ear serves as a reminder of our prenatal conditions. The Chinese Taoists claim that they can transform grey hair back to its natural color after a certain amount of time spent performing these breathing techniques. They even claim that they can grow back lost teeth or missing limbs. Personally I feel that ignorant as we are in the mechanism of creation, this may be possible. There are forms of animal life capable of such regeneration, which proves that this process is not alien to our world.

In Buddhist philosophy the ears only represent one lotus, of which there are many all over the body, in the important centers of interrelationship with the Cosmos, or Divine Mother. There are lotuses at the top of the head, on the forehead, eyes, nose, chest, abdomen, palms of the hands, feet, etc., as represented in the frontispiece. Each petal of the lotus represents a meridian or organic function. At the same time it represents a psychic function. Thus the acupuncture point Pai Hui, or TM 20,* which means 100 union point (situated at the top of the head), is the same as the Hindu Shakra by the name of 1000 petal lotus. The Chinese figure of 100 is symbolic of the infinite amount of awarenesses that is opened up and channelled through this point of higher mental processes. At the same time the four extra points around TM 20, named the 4 Gods or Heavenly Stars, are the same as the 4 Gurus at the top of the head in Hindu philosophy.

---

*See abreviation table on page 191

To get back specifically to the ear, Chinese physiology uses it to examine the state of our ancestral energy (Yuan Qi). The ear is the external flowering of the kidneys and they are directly connected by an internal meridian. (When we cannot find adequate scientific explanation, we must resort to the traditional Chinese viewpoint as the modern Chinese do.)

The kidneys are the organs which store this ancestral energy, given to us at the time of conception and accompanying us till death. It is this basic energy which gives us our strength and vitality, without which we would be dead at birth (which is often the case), and which food, drink and oxygen serve to nourish. When the post-natal or principal meridians are affected, the disease is not as complicated as when the prenatal meridians are affected.

THE ROLE OF EAR ACUPUNCTURE IN THE WEST

Ear acupuncture is effective in numerous diseases, and particularly in controlling pain. In operations done under acupuncture analgesia it is the ear points which are most important and a great number of operations are done using only ear points. There seems to be a transmission of the ear loci stimulation to the thalamus, or pain controlling centres and thence to the cerebral cortex. (Note this is only a tentative explanation.)

Ear acupuncture can play a leading role in North America as a quick, inexpensive and simple treatment of the drug and alcohol addiction rampant here. Experiments of this nature have been carried out successfully in Kwong Wah and Tung Wah hospitals in Hong Kong and recently in the U.S.A. The patient is completely free and disintoxicated, as proven by various tests, within 60 days after inception of treatment.

CHAPTER 3

STRUCTURE OF THE EXTERNAL EAR (AURICLE)

If we look closely at the ear we realize that it is also shaped like a funnel. Needless to say, this funnel serves the purpose of collecting and directing soundwaves to the brain. The screening of the sound waves does not begin at the eardrums, but actually much before. The various ridges and irregularities of the ear have already made a primary selection of different qualities of sound waves, which are accordingly directed towards the auditory canal where a more intensive selection is elaborated at the tympanic membrane. Therefore the auricle serves as a primary radar screen which first captures sound waves on its sensitive cells and divides these waves into Yin (—) and Yang (+) waves. The positive and negative waves are set into motion in clockwise and counterclockwise directions and as they approach the tympanum their gyrations increase in intensity and are funnelled internally where a further selection and distribution takes place. I am emitting the hypothesis, therefore, that the shape, structure and texture of the external ear determines the quality of the sound waves we receive.

What then is the texture of the auricle? It is built up mostly of cartilage, connective tissue and fat. These "fabrics" are irrigated and activated by a large amount of blood vessels, nerve endings and lymph glands directly beneath the skin. To describe the structure more readily according to the function I have described in the previous paragraph, it would be easier to take point 0, or central point of the ear, as shown in diagram 2, as the point of reference.

We then notice that the ear forms a series of concentric ridges about point "0" and that there is a sort of appendage hanging at the bottom which consists mainly of fatty tissue (ear lobe, or lobule). The area immediately surrounding point "0" is concave anteriorly and contains the passage (auditory meatus) leading to the inner ear and the inside of the skull. Let us say that this is the courtyard of the castle, (to keep in the frame of mind of Chinese medicine,), and the canal is the tunnel leading to the Royal suite, or Chambers (brain). The area on the posterior of the auricle corresponding to this one is convex and if one looks at it objectively, it resembles a fireman's helmet. It is separated from the base of the skull by a vertical ridge. Muscles join this area to the skull, giving the ears some mobility. Since, however, man does not have as much voluntary control over his ears as do most animals, he sometimes has to push his ear forward with his hand at the back of the ear to better capture the sound waves.

Again, if one compares the ear to a micro-castle, the rim (helix) of the ear represents the exterior fortification, or wall, and extends along the whole border of the ear in the form of a question mark to the lobule. As far as the lobule is concerned this does not have to be fortified since it consists of fatty tissue, which has a sinking quality, or sliding quality, comparable to swamp or quicksand and the enemy can only slip or sink in this area.

Within this first wall there is another concentric ridge, or inner wall, separated from the first by a depression which resembles the moat of a castle. Toward the top of the ear this ridge divides in two parts and contains a triangular depression, which we can compare to a secret radar or armament station within the castle.

My reason for describing the ear in so poetic a fashion is to welcome you to the ear, and make it your ally and associate. An ally always responds better when something of the heart is put into the relationship. I believe Chinese medical philosophy to be a refined form of poetry, for the purpose of making the laws of nature the allies of the doctor.

I will now go on to describe each part of the auricle. (Diagram 2.)

DIAGRAM 2
Structure of the Auricle

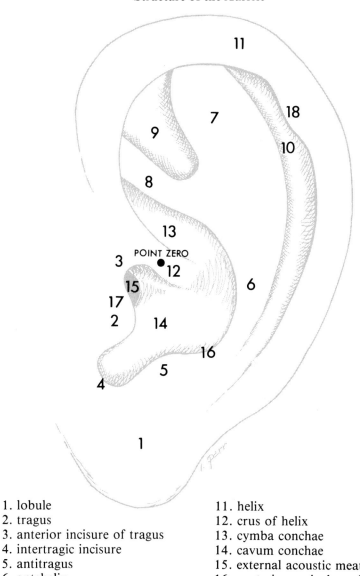

1. lobule
2. tragus
3. anterior incisure of tragus
4. intertragic incisure
5. antitragus
6. antehelix
7. upper crura of antehelix
8. lower crura of antehelix
9. triangular fossa
10. scaphoid fossa
11. helix
12. crus of helix
13. cymba conchae
14. cavum conchae
15. external acoustic meatus
16. posterior auricular sulcus
17. tuberculum supratragicum
18. auricular (Darwin's) tubercle
19. posterior auricle

1) **Lobule:** A soft, fatty appendage at the bottom of the auricle, making up 1/4 to 1/5 of its length on the average.

2) **Tragus:** A cartilagineous projection jutting out over the auditory canal or meatus, to protect it.

3) **Anterior Incisure of Tragus:** Separates the tragus from the crus of the helix above it.

4) **Intertragic Incisure:** A notch at the bottom of the tragus, separating it from the antitragus, a projection on the top of the lobule.

5) **Antitragus:** A projection at the top of the lobule, opposite the tragus, at the lower end of the anthelix, or inner wall of the fortification. If one were to further draw a similarity to a snake, the anthelix would form the tail end and the antitragus the head of the snake.

6) **Anthelix:** The tail end of the above mentioned snake, divided superiorly into two branches or forks of the snake's tail. It forms a semi-circular ridge about the auditory meatus and comprises the inner wall of the above mentioned castle.

7) **Upper Crura (root) of Anthelix:** The upper branch of the tail division of the snake.

8) **Lower Crura (root) of Anthelix:** The lower branch of the tail end of the snake formed by the anthelix.

9) **Triangular Fossa:** The triangular depression formed between the upper and lower crurae of the anthelix.

10) **Scaphoid Fossa:** The depression or mote between the helix and anthelix.

11) **Helix:** Inverted rim of the auricle, shaped like a question mark without the dot.

12) **Crus (root) of helix:** The root of the helix, where the latter attaches itself to the concave depression about the auditory meatus.

13) **Cymba Conchae:** The superior part of the concavity (concha) above the crus of the helix.

14) **Cavum Conchae:** The inferior part of the concavity (concha) below the crus of the helix, containing the auditory canal. Together both conchae form the concha.

15) **External Acoustic Meatus:** The external auditory canal, situated in the cavum conchae, and protected exteriorly by the tragus.

16) **Posterior Auricular Sulcus:** The notch separating the anthelix from the antitragus.

17) **Tuberculum Supratragicum:** A small projection over the tragus, limited superiorly by the insisure of the tragus.

18) **Auricular (Darwin's) Tubercle:** A small projection on the free margin of the helix, facing the anthelix.

19) **Posterior Auricle:** The back of the ear, the convex portion.

VASCULARIZATION AND INNERVATION OF THE EXTERNAL EAR (AURICLE) (Diagram 3)

a) **Arteries:** The arterial vascularization of the ala auris (wing of the ear, or auricle) is ensured by the superficial temporal and posterior auricular branches of the external carotid artery.

b) **Veins:** The veins of the auricle drain either into the superficial temporal vein anteriorly, or into the external jugular vein and mastoid vein posteriorly.

c) **Lymphatics:** There are three groups of lymphatics in the auricle:

—anterior group: drains into the pretragic lymph nodes.

—posterior group: drains into the mastoid and posterior auricular lymph nodes.

—inferior group: drains into the parotid lymph nodes.

d) **Nerves:** There is an abundant nerve supply in the auricle which derive from the facial nerve, trigeminal, glossopharyngeal, vagus, major and minor occipital nerves. They can be subdivided into two types: motor nerves and sensitive nerves.

The motor nerves are ramifications of the nervus facialis. Its temporal branch activates the anterior auricular muscles, the superior auricular muscles and the frontal muscles.

The sensitive nerves are extended from the auriculotemporal nerve of the lower mandible and the auricular branch of the superificial cervical plexus. Among the sensitive nerves of the anterior auricle we find branches of the trigeminal nerve, from which a branch of the trochlear and supraorbital nerves spread out to the anterior cranial region. A zygomaticotemporal branch spreads out to the anterior temporal region. A third, auriculotemporal branch spreads out to the lateral cranial region of the ear and to the opening of the external auditory meatus.

The posterior auricular sensitive nerves derive from the cervical plexus. The major auricular nerve and minor occipital nerve course superficially along the sternocleidomastoideus muscle and reach the bottom of the face and the inferior and posterior auricular areas. The major auricular nerve splits at the lobule into anterior and posterior branches which reach different areas of the auricle.

The vagus nerve extends to the posterior auricular region and to the inferior wall of the external auditory meatus.

Thus we can see that different parts of the auricle, such as the scapha, lobule, triangular fossa, helix, etc, are innervated by branches of different nerves. Consequently it can be deduced that a stimulation of one area of the ear sends a message to a different part of the body than a stimulation at another point or area. At the same time since nerve endings belong to different nerves are found quite close to each other on the auricle, this may explain why we can find for instance a Knee point 2mm. away from a Heart point. I must point out however, that all the nerves in the ear have not yet been traced and that Chinese medicine does not claim to function according to nervous meridians alone.

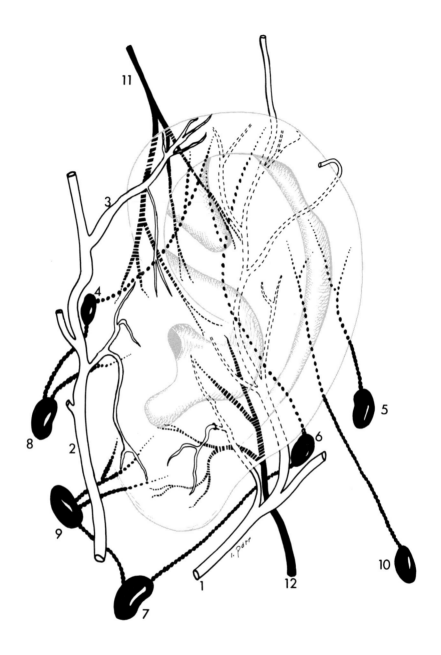

DIAGRAM 3
Vascularization & Innervation of the Auricle

1. Occipital artery
2. Superficial temporal artery
3. Anterior auricular artery
4. Pretragic lymph node
5. Mastoid lymph node
6. Posterior auricular lymph node
7. Parotid lymph node
8., 9. Anterior auricular lymph nodes
10. Spinal lymph node
11. Auriculotemporal nerve
12. Auricular branch of the
     superficial cervical plexus

SECTION II:

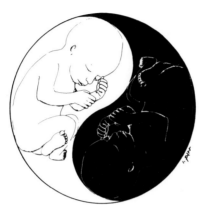

Diagnosis & Technique

CHAPTER **4**

EXAMINING THE PATIENT

This is by far the most important step before applying the needles. I know of many neophytes in acupuncture who overlook this step and are anxious to just needle people anywhere. This is analagous to being a guest in someone's house and jumping for the cake and throwing away the meal. Morever here in North America I have heard and seen prominent doctors purport to teach shortcuts in the field of acupuncture. Needless to say, not only will the results be few, but not many patients will return to you for their subsequent treatments, especially now that the "Craze of Acupuncture" has practically disappeared and that the public is becoming wary of "farcers."

To quote my professor, Master Lok Yee-Kung:

"A dead person does not need treatment. One must be careful and attentive when dealing with human life. People come to you because they are sick. You are in the position of a tiger, but you must not maul the people, you must examine them gently with the smoothness of a pussycat."

The following types of diagnosis are to be applied to all forms of acupuncture, ear acupuncture included. Though the technique is somewhat different in that it deals exclusively with the ear, the human body is the same and we are still within the scope of Chinese medicine. With respect to diagnosis, Chinese techniques are not altogether different from Western medical techniques in as far as common sense is concerned. The West has the sole advantage of possessing X-rays and labs, which though often helpful, just as often are not.

There are four basic procedures in diagnosing a patient, which are as follows:

1) Wang: by Inspection (observation)

The external appearance of the patient is examined. This procedure begins as soon as he walks through the door . . . . Does he enter in a brusque movement, slamming the door? Does he walk in shyly, hesitatingly? Does he stand straight, stooped? Does he limp?

How does he dress? Regardless of price of clothing, is he neat, sloppy? Are both shoes the same? Is his hair messy? . . . What are his manners like? . . . What colors is he wearing? Is there a preference of color to be determined from one treatment to the next? All this is important as colors are directly related to the states of the internal organs. For example, a person with poor blood circulation might prefer red, one with liver or stomach problems blue, green or yellow.

It is most often these very first impressions that the doctor receives, from the moment the patient enters his office, that are the clues to his ailment and condition. Further tests only help to verify what the first observations found out.

The famous Dr. Bell of England, who was Conan Doyle's medical teacher, and whose techniques inspired the latter to write "Sherlock Holmes", used his waiting room as an observation unit and most of his amazingly precise diagnoses were made right there.

Then we get into particulars, such as the face, voice, skin coloration, urine and stool coloration, etc.

What type of facial expression does the patient have? Does he look happy, sad, melancholic? Is his expression one of pain? This is usually indicative of a recent or acute disorder. Does he have a weak and drowsy look, possibly indicating a chronic, long-abused state? Is his face deep red, a sign of fever or high blood pressure? Is he pale, indicating a possible anemia or internal hemorrhaging?

Does he keep his head bent to one side? This may be due to muscular atrophy, vitamin deficiency or a spinal subluxation.

Is his forehead wrinkled? This is a worrier. Does he have small verticle wrinkles inbetween the eyebrows? This is a common sign of liver trouble of some sort. Are there small venal stasis on either cheek, possibly indicating pulmonary or hepatic deficiency?

Then there is the examination of the tongue which plays as an important role in Chinese medicine as in Western medicine. The Chinese divide the tongue into different regions, each corresponding to a particular organ. The coloring and coating of the tongue is likewise ascribed to specific disorders. This information may be found in most translations of "The Yellow Emperor's Classic of Internal Medicine", the Nei Ching.

2) Wen: by Listening

This type of examination consists of listening to see the quality of the patient's voice. A strong smooth voice usually indicates a good resistance to disease, whereas a weak voice indicates a poor resistance. The pitch, frequency, resonance, are all taken into consideration. The doctor listens to the complaints of the patient attentively, without interrupting. The smell of body odors is also noted.

3) Wun: by Inquiry

The patient is then asked about the situation which led to his ailment, about his social condition, family life, possible hereditary factors, types of previous treatments and results, etc.

4) Tse: by Palpation (pulse)

The pulse is then examined as to regularity of beats, amplitude, texture, and so on as in ordinary acupuncture. Various areas of the body are palpated to check for pain referral and tension, such as the abdominal area, neck, and areas of complaint.

The above examination should precede every treatment and the pulse taken after every treatment as well. Usually it will be found that the pulse will appear entirely different in quality, depending on whether the treatment administered was correct or not.

CONTRA-INDICATIONS TO
EAR ACUPUNCTURE THERAPY

Although most diseases can be treated with success by ear acupuncture, there are some important precautions to take with regard to specific exceptions.

a) Ear acupuncture, just as ordinary acupuncture, should not be administered to weak, tired, hungry people, or those who have not completely digested their meal, or who are under the influence of alcohol.

b) One should refrain from applying ear acupuncture to pregnant women, especially during the first five months of pregnancy, as this may cause premature delivery, or abortion. After this initial period, ear acupuncture may be administered for the alleviation of pain. Great care must be taken not to needle certain points, such as the uterus, ovary, internal secretion, pelvis and abdomen points. There is, however, a treatment classically applied with ordinary acupuncture which may prove beneficial with ear treatment. The Ki 9 locus, if needled twice during pregnancy, alone, is reputed to have the property to erase bad hereditary traits from both parents and allow the child to begin an entirely free cycle of existence with such benefits as exceptional health and longevity. Experiments to confirm this theory have been carried out in France for about 30 years and appear to confirm it. As far as longevity is concerned we have no definite proof, since the research is too recent. However, those children whose mothers received this treatment appear extremely healthy, with fresh rosy cheeks, and should they become ill, the condition never persists more than a couple of days. I have tried it once personally on a woman the doctors considered unhealthy and too weak to bear a healthy child, if at all. She gave birth to an exceptionally healthy child with a head full of hair and rosy cheeks, much to everyone's astonishment. Of course this may be pure coincidence. Perhaps your experiments in this area may prove the theory correct 100 years from now!

c) Anemic people should generally not be treated by ear acupuncture, unless this appears to be a last resort. The patient must be warned of possible risks of fainting, dizziness or nausea. In such cases permanent press-needles are more suitable as they provide a milder and more gradual stimulation. These needles shall be described later.

d) Nervous or weak patients should always be allowed to lie down for a period up to one half hour prior to treatment, and following treatment. Quite often these patients may say that they feel fine after the treatment and then faint once they go out into the street. It is recommended to offer them a glass of warm water, or Chinese tea to draw back energy into the triple burners, which will stimulate recuperation.

e) Old people should be allowed to rest before and after application of the needles, especially if ear blood-letting techniques are used, such as is commonly the case with arteriosclerosis or high blood pressure. Great care must be taken not to take more than 2-3 drops from a point, which is quite sufficient to lead to an improvement of the condition. Also, no more than one or two points should be bled per treatment. Chinese bleeding techniques have nothing in common with the primitive blood-letting applied by our barbers not very long ago.

f) Extremely old and weak patients should not be needled until there is some improvement of their condition. This can be done in several ways:
—by massaging the ears with the fingers during a series of 10-15 treatments.
—by stimulating the ear points 2-3 minutes at a time with the end of a matchstick or probe (smooth), during a series of treatment.
—by applying 'moxa' to certain body points such as Ho-ku large intestine 4. and San-li, Stomach 36, and Ren Mo 4, 6, 12, Tu Mo 4. This technique will be explained later.

The patient will be judged ready to undergo "needle therapy" according to improvement in skin coloration, blood-pressure, weight, digestion, improved sleeping, mobility, etc.

g) Young children of less than 7 years of age usually should not be needled. This is due to their lack of sufficient energetic stability and growth. Again in such cases, massage may be employed, or else small permanent press-needles, or ion-spheres* or seeds may be used. The latter may be applied to the ear points, covered with a band-aid and maintained in place for several days up to one week. The child's parents should be told to rub them gently for 2-3 minutes at a time several times during the day. Great care must be taken to avoid infection or "shrivelling" of the ears. Wetting the ears while these needles are in place should also be avoided. In the case of infection, the patient should return immediately to the doctor who will apply some penecillin ointment (unless allergic) or other disinfectant or antibiotic.

N.B.: Certain points have the property of combatting infection. These are: Suprarenal Gland, Kidney, Outer Ear and Occiput points.

h) A patient who walks in from the cold, or who is suffering from frost-bite, or inflammation of the ears should not be treated immediately. The temperature of the ears must first be restored to normal, or the inflammation brought down, either by waiting, as in less severe cases, or by needling the suprarenal gland, kidney, occiput and outer ear points to restore the ear to its normal condition. (Rubbing the ear, in the case of cold ears.)

i) Permanent press-needles should not be used in warm weather, as chances of infection are greater at this time.

ACUPUNCTURE INTOLERANCE

Certain patients may present what is usually referred to as "acupuncture intolerance syndrome". After application of needles, certain reactions occur, such as dizziness, fainting, numbness of limbs, head-ache, cold sweat, nausea, a high drop in blood-pressure, or extreme pain in the body or helix of the auricle.

If the symptoms are mild, merely talking to the patient will restore the balance, by reassuring him that nothing serious is happening. In extremely severe cases, however, the needles should

---

*Ion-spheres: minute metal balls which can be applied to the surface of the skin and covered with a bandage, to produce a mild and gradual stimulation of the points.

either be withdrawn immediately and the patient's head lowered to restore blood circulation, or the needles merely released slightly, but not entirely withdrawn. Otherwise, needling the suprarenal gland, dermis, heart and occiput points, or He 9 on the tip of the little finger will bring recovery.

The physician need not be alarmed by these reactions. He must remain calm and collected at all times. The proof that there is nothing serious to worry about is that the symptoms disappear immediately once the needles are slightly withdrawn and in any case rarely last more than a couple of minutes. Some warm tea may be offered the patient once he feels a little better.

Such reactions are usually due to too deep insertion of the needles, a stimulation which is too strong for that particular patient, or too many needles. Quite often upon interrogating the patient afterwards you will find that he did not eat for several hours prior to the treatment, or he hadn't slept well or not at all the night before, or was taking a drug that you were not told about. Perhaps it was only a nervous reaction due to too much absorption of coffee or tea before the treatment, or alcohol. These reactions are often positive as they oblige the physician to delve down more deeply into the patient's personal habits and elicit the complete truth from him. How many patients lie to their doctors from fear of being reprimanded?

The Proper Position to Treat the Patient

It is best to treat the patient in a horizontal position, laying him down on a comfortable bed or table which is at a convenient height so that the person treating can examine and apply the needles without having to bend too much. The acupuncturist can sit in a chair, at the head of the bed. The comfort of both patient and doctor is not to be overlooked, as this largely determines a correct diagnosis, needle application and serves to reassure the patient that he can have faith in whoever is treating him.

To begin the examination of the ear itself the doctor places his chair at the head of the table or bed, behind the patient's head. He can then go on to feel both ears between the index and thumb of both hands to check for irregularities of texture, shape, temperature. By moving the chair slightly to either side he can examine the ears individually, by touch and with a magnifying glass. What it is exactly that he is looking for shall be discussed in a later chapter dealing with diagnosis. It is wise to have a stencil copy of the ear handy to jot down the precise loci which present abnormalities.

EXAMINING THE EARS

Upon examining the ears there are several steps to take:

1) **Palpating the ears:** Both ears are palpated between the index finger and thumbs in order to try to identify any irregularities in shape or form. One may begin at the lobule and work one's way up and around, onto the back of the ears. Any irregularities such as bumps, lumps, abcesses, slippery feeling, coarseness, granular feeling, peeling, should be noted and jotted onto the schematic ear representation which should be kept in the file.

2) **Looking:** This is best done with a magnifying glass. One should note any discoloration or different coloration than in surrounding areas. Sometimes a point may appear whiter, grayer, redder than the area next to it.

3) **Painful spots:** These may be sought by applying slight to hard pressure all about the ear until pain is expressed by the patient. One may use the end of a matchstick, a metal probe or directly with the end of the needle, to locate this painful spot.

In general, when using the end of the needle to check for pain, one must be careful not to insert the needle deeply. A mere pecking action with the needle is sufficient. The advantage of using the needle instead of the probe or matchstick is obvious when we are dealing with such a small surface area as the ear presents to us and when the points are so close together. The needle tip presents an extremely small surface area and by pecking around a locus one may locate the precise area of the point where the pain is greatest. Otherwise it is difficult to know if you are right on the point or on its edge. As you know an acupuncture point on the ear has a radius of 1-2 mm. but it is the centre of the point which is deemed most effective in affecting relief of symptoms and a cure.

4) **Insensitive spots:** Certain loci, even when a very hard pressure is exerted, compared to the area immediately adjacent, show no reaction at all. One must differentiate between this type of reaction and that of certain patients who do not react to pain at all (stoics). This is a pathological condition which can be verified by checking the corresponding peripheral area on the body which will usually likewise show a hypoanalgesic reaction, bearing witness to a functional disorder due to many causes which need be determined.

5) **Cold sensitivity test:** The purpose of this test is to identify which points on the ear, if any, do not react to a stimulation by a freezing probe. If such is the case, it is indicative of peripheral vasoconstrictive disorders in the corresponding area of the body. Again this can be verified immediately by say, if it is the hip point which presents this type of reaction, the skin on the surface of the hip will most likely appear cold to the touch. By mobilizing the hip there is usually a correction of this state and the ear locus likewise regains normality and reacts positively to the cold probe.

To obtain such a cold probe, one may insert a needle in a metal pen cap which is placed in a saucer containing ice-cubes. One must be careful not to wet the needle as this would alter the nature of the findings.

6) **Heat sensitivity test:** For this test the needle must be quite hot. It is not easy to maintain the heat for more than several seconds before it cools down. One may have a burning moxa cigar close at hand (to be described later), which maintains a steady and intensive heat of several hundred degrees at its centre, and put the end of the needle in contact with it. A piece of tape can be rolled around the other end (handle) of the needle to protect the fingers from being burned. If the patient does not feel the heat of the needle, this is generally indicative of a peripheral vasodilation in the corresponding area of the body, bearing symptoms such as neuralgia, high temperature, inflammation, or rheumatism. In this type of case, the condition is made worse by massage,

mobilization or manipulation, whereas in the previous test, massage and mobilization tended to improve the condition.

7) **Pulse:** The pulse should be taken before, immediately after and at the end of the treatment. Many ear acupuncture specialists prefer to palpate the radial artery with the thumb during the entire process of applying the needles. This method has definite advantages in that one knows immediately which needle has the greatest reaction on the patient (positive or negative). Although every needle applied is important, in that they prepare the terrain, it is usually one single needle which causes the greatest reaction and affects the cure. When using this technique, one must wait several seconds to check for a reaction before inserting the following needle. This reaction is either an acceleration of the beat rhythm immediately or after a few seconds, likewise it can be a diminishing of the rhythm immediately, or after a few seconds, or else it may be an apparent halt of the pulse with a normalization following. Once any of the above reactions have been noted the patient should be interrogated as to how he now feels compared to before. If there is an improvement, one need no longer apply subsequent needles. Another advantage of this method over simply applying the needles according to painful spots and pathology formulae is the close contact that the physician maintains with the patient, which unscientific as it may seem, nevertheless serves to improve his condition. The psychological factor, though it may represent no more than 20% of the curing effect, is nevertheless important to consider. Likewise, if the symptoms are aggravated by a certain needle, the physician will know immediately which one it is. Quite often the condition does appear to be aggravated after a certain needle has been applied. It is wise not to withdraw the needle immediately but to wait a few seconds as, just as often, the patient will state that he feels much better after and that he no longer feels many, if not all, of his symptoms. This is because the stimulation caused a general acceleration of his metabolism and led to a recovery.

8) **Precautions:** In the above steps, great care must be taken to use only extreme reactions as reference for treatment. These are extreme reactions to heat and cold, extreme reactions to pain. They are interpreted by the patient's jumping, grimacing, painful contortion of the face, or yelling. However, some patients tend to

exaggerate and are provoked to jump at the slightest touch. In their mind, the mere fact of undergoing a medical examination is synonymous to obvious pain. It is wise to double check the findings after five to ten minutes, as they may prove to be very different from the first. In the case of very old or weak people, great care must be taken not to examine them too intensely at a time, since the various responses that you are looking for may prove to be too strong a stimulation with subsequent complications arising.

Still other people may show no reaction to pain although in fact they may be experiencing it at an intolerable level. Such people may either be stoics, or else they may be anticipating drastic measure taken by the doctor should they admit the pain. For this purpose it is often useful to use an electrical devise for the detection of pain.

9) **Electronic Detection:** Various types of electronic devices for the detection of pain are available on the market, either of French, Chinese, Japanese, Canadian or American origin. These machines work on the principle that acupuncture points are areas of the skin having a lower resistance to electrical currents and therefore of higher conductivity. They are equipped with a mass electrode which the patient holds in his hand and an electrode attached to a search probe which is passed over the surface of the ear to locate the pathological points.

When a point is located, this is verified either by an indicator on a meter, by a small bulb which is lit up or by a buzz or a bell which can be heard. In the latter case the auditory effect is increased or diminished according to the intensity of the pain at the ear loci. Some of these instruments contain all of the above mechanisms, which makes them more practical and precise. Before using any of these devises, a few of which I shall describe, it is important to dry the ear with 95% alcohol and clean it so as to obviate the humidity factor which alters the findings. Sometimes this has to be done during the detection as well, as the texture of the skin of the auricle can change during the process of detection.

Another advantage of this type of examination, besides the obvious objective aspect, is that it is less time consuming than the other methods and at the same time most machines are equipped with different types of currents that can be applied spontaneously to the ear points without the needle. These currents need not be applied more than several seconds in most cases but can be maintained up to ten minutes in more difficult or severe conditions. Also the fact that the most recent ones have a highly sensitive spring attached to the end of the search probe, leads to a more precise detection of the points and eliminates the patient's pain during detection, as is the case in the other methods, since the pressure exerted need not be felt by the patient.

In patients that are "wary" of the needle, or in children, the spontaneous application of currents is highly beneficial.

a) **Nogier's Therapuncteur:** This apparatus can be either battery operated or branched to a wall socket. It emits positive, negative or alternating square wave currents of an intensity of 80—100 micro-amps under 60 volts. Its rhythm is about one hertz, which is similar to the cardiac rhythm.

Its probes are designed to treat either large areas at once or minute spots. It differs from other machines in that the current applied in the case of a stimulation passes only through the acupuncture point and does not continue through the neck and arm as is the case with the hand ground mass in most devices. This allows the effects of the treatment to be appreciated to the stimulation of a precise locus and not to a larger area of the body.

b) **Pellin's Stigmascope:** It contains 18-V batteries which can be recharged. A small red light warns us of weakened batteries. The patient holds the ground mass in his hand and the negative electrode is attached to the probe. As the probe approaches the vacinity of the point, a warning sound is given which increases in intensity as the point is precisely detected. At the same time, a light tells us that we are approaching a point. The acoustic device will emit varying pitches of sound according to the degree of pathological aggravation of the locus.

A list of various electronic devices readily available on the market here and the addresses where they can be purchased, are given in the Appendix I. No doubt far better devises shall be developed in the very near future, as even these have a very short history.

10) **Absence of pain referral:** There are a great deal of patients whose ears do not present any painful spots although

those same patients are obviously suffering. In Chinese terms this would be explained by stating that there is a lack of "Chi (Qi)" (vital energy) arriving at the ears and that this "Chi" is blocked further down along the ear channel and does not express itself exteriorly. There are several steps to take in order to bring about the pain referral to the surface of the ear. One may either rub the auricle itself, or the lobule to bring about this response. One may use moxa or infra-red rays. Or else, certain stimulating points which have the property of "opening" the ear are needled, such as Shen Men, Diaphragm, or Point Zero.

Another method consists of rubbing the area on the body that the patient is complaining about for a few minutes. Very often this will succeed in bringing about a response in the ear. Naturally, it would be wiser to combine several of these methods at once so as not to waste time, such as rubbing the auricle or lobule with the fingers or a matchstick, needling the Diaphragm point, and rubbing the ailing part of the body, and afterwards proceeding to apply the regular ear treatment.

However there are still cases that do not respond even to this sort of preparation. In such cases, simply needling the points on the auricle that correspond to their particular ailment will bring about a cure.

11) **Homolaterality or contralaterality of certain points:** Although Stomach, Spleen, Liver and Heart points exist on both auricles, these organs are generally best treated by the homolateral ear. One exception is the Lungs. There are two lung points on either ear. Of the two, the lower point corresponds to the lung on the same side and the upper point to the opposite lung.

Generally speaking, the aforementioned points included, about 80% of all patients have homolateral reactions to the ear points. The remaining 20% react contralaterally. How can this be determined effectively? Actually it is very difficult. It is often easier to just needle both ears. Only the effective point will react to the stimulation. If one uses the pulse technique mentioned just previously, this can be somewhat obviated, as the reaction to each point is noted on the pulse. Though this does prevent unnecessary needling of too many points, it does not indicate which side to needle on. One of my colleagues has developed an interesting technique which many of us have found successful to date. The patient is told to lie down flat on his stomach and after a few minutes to turn over on his back. If he crosses his legs upon turning over, 90% of the time this is a sign of contralateral reactions to ear points in general and even to body points.

Most often, one will not find the same pathological points on both ears. This is normal for several reasons. First of all, no one's ears are the same on both sides, and secondly, if a person is suffering in a certain part of the body, only the corresponding side receives pain referral signals in 80% of all cases. Therefore one need needle only the points on the same side most of the time. There are techniques which stress the importance of needling one or two points on the opposite ear as well in order to direct an excess of energy on one side of the body to the other side for easier elimination of toxins and to relieve the affected side.

PRECAUTIONS TO TAKE
IN NEEDLING THE EAR

No two people experience exactly the same emotions, pain, nor are they constructed in exactly the same way. Ear acupuncture takes this into consideration, just as does ordinary acupuncture. Quite often the needle is put into the same point in different patients. This appears to be relatively simple. However, the fact is that the needle is not inserted in exactly the same way from one patient to the other. The contact of the needle to the skin is never exactly the same. Methods of needling vary from patient to patient.

One may compare the patient to a guitar. I'm sure many of you are familiar to this comparison, which is classical at this point, just as has become the comparison of a human being to a car. I prefer the guitar as I find it more harmonious to the human soul . . . . No two guitars are out of tune in exactly the same way. To tune it, one must tighten this string a little, loosen the other one more or less . . . until one succeeds in reaching the desired state of harmony. This is established according to some sort of statistics which are, in the case of the guitar, your scale of notes and harmonies.

In acupuncture, or medicine, they are blood pressure, color of eyes, weight, muscle tone, sleeping habits, etc. All in all, whether we are speaking about a guitar or a human being, what we are looking for is discordant notes which have a "sour" pitch according to our scales. We are trained to observe in a certain way. We might add that as far as medicine is concerned, the Occident has invented the major scale and the Orient the minor scale. Both can be married for the benefit of mankind.

This is why, when we are told to needle such and such a point for such and such a disease, this may be quite right. The important thing to remember however, is how to apply the needle to different points and to different patients. Some people must be practically stabbed (not from arms length of course), others must be pecked with the needle, still others must have the needle twisted one way or the other, and in others the needle is slanted at various angles. These are techniques which are perfected only through experience, and by observation at the hands of a master. When I began to learn acupuncture, I was obliged to spend three months performing various exercises to loosen my wrists. Although I found this to be a highly sophisticated form of "Chinese torture" at the time, I am indeed grateful to my teachers for this now.

Sterilization: Before applying the needles they must be thoroughly sterilized. The entire surface of the auricle, back, front, and hidden regions must be cleansed with a cotton ball dipped in 75% alcohol. 75% alcohol is more recommended than 95% since its water content allows it to penetrate deeper than pure alcohol. If an infection should occur after needling, those areas should be cleansed with 2.5% iodine or penecillin gauze (except for allergic reactions). Otherwise one may needle the Outer Ear, Suprarenal Gland, Occiput and Kidney points, which have the property of stimulating the defenses of the organism and thereby combatting infection.

How to Insert the Needle: The procedure is described for a right handed person. A left handed person would apply the opposite hand in the same way. The thumb and index finger of the left hand are supporting the auricle, with the index finger behind the auricle to make sure the needle doesn't penetrate to the other side. The thumb stretches the area about the point, to ensure precision in needling. This also helps to reduce pain and to calm the patient. Some people just jab the ear without touching the patient. I find the laying on of hands, so to speak, quite benefitial.

CHAPTER 5

The needle is then inserted rapidly with the thumb and index finger of the right hand, either directly, or with a twist. By twisting the needle upon insertion, a greater stimulation is provided and obviates the necessity of further twisting after the needle is in place. For a hyperactive (Yang) patient the needle is twisted to the left, or counterclockwise, for a hypoactive (Yin) patient the needle is twisted to the right, or clockwise.

The needle must be imbedded firmly in the cartilage or whatever area is needled in order to produce a curing effect. A sloppy and superficial needle will produce no effect at all.

The amount of time the needle is left in place may vary from two minutes to 1/2 hour, remaining as long as 1-2 hours in patients suffering from chronic conditions. Quite often, the patient will feel an improvement immediately after insertion. The needle may then be removed and the patient given another appointment in no later than 7 days. On the average 20 minutes is deemed necessary and sufficient.

Often, a small very thin tack-like needle is used. This type of needle can be left in place for several days, up to one week, and covered with a bandage to prevent it from falling out. This type of needle is beneficial for chronic sufferers who can not come for treatment every day, for old people, children, and drug addicts. They are told to rub the needles for a few minutes several times during the day. Great care must be taken to avoid infection with these needles, as the cartilage has no defences, and the patient must be warned not to wet them while taking a shower, or to return immediately on the slightest sign of infection. In very warm weather, chances of infection are greater, therefore this type of treatment is not to be applied.

There are other similar methods utilizing take-home techniques. Instead of the needle small metal balls called ion-spheres, or small seeds can be attached to the ear points and covered with a band-aid and left in place just as the tack or permanent needles. Again this is beneficial for children who are too young to be needled, for hypersensitive adults, or for old people.

Frequency of treatment: Research done in mainland China deems it necessary to administer three series of ten treatments each at daily intervals, interspaced by one week to allow the organism to rest and recover on its own. In Europe and America, one treatment a week is found to be sufficient, although no more than one week should elapse between at least the first three or four treatments.

It is quite possible that the Chinese obtain better results by giving more treatments at closer intervals, however this is difficult to apply in the North American or European context, both from the doctor's point of view and from the patient's for obvious reasons. I should recommend therefore that chronic sufferers be allowed 2-3 treatments a week for several weeks and recent or not as complicated conditions be allotted one treatment per week. If a patient finds improvement immediately after the first treatment, he can usually be set back one to two weeks immediately. Quite often also, it may be found that such patients, upon returning for their second treatment will complain that during the week the pain returned as badly as before and that they have not improved in the slightest. Upon close examination, checking the mobility, or inflammation, or whatever the case may be, the doctor will usually find some sort of improvement, no matter how slight it may appear. The third week the patient may again complain that he has no improvement, though again a closer look will prove otherwise. These are normal reactions which are eliminated right after the session and return during the week. They usually last no more than three treatments. Should they last longer, than say 4 or 5 treatments, the physician may continue to treat the patient at the risk of soiling his reputation as an extortionist who is only interested in money, or he may tell the patient to return in a few months. The seasons have a large influence in diseases and it happens quite often that certain patients who did not respond at all during one season, react marvelously during another. This is due to the evolutionary and devolutionary peaks of every individual. In Chinese philosophy this is very well explained with the cycles of what is termed as the "10 Heavenly Stems and the 12 Earthly Branches". According to this system certain patients should not be treated on certain days. This is similar to the biorhythm methods which have been developed in modern times and widely applied in many countries.

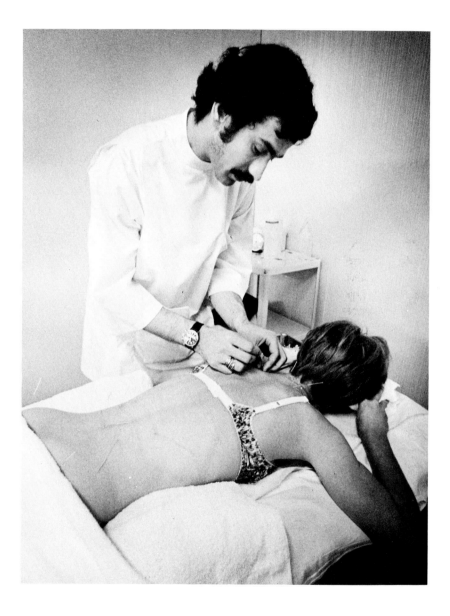

Author treating a patient.

DIAGRAM 4
Needling techniques

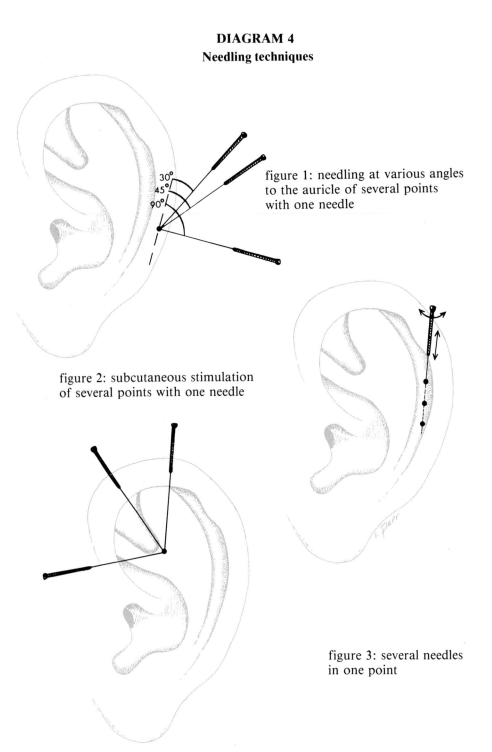

figure 1: needling at various angles
to the auricle of several points
with one needle

figure 2: subcutaneous stimulation
of several points with one needle

figure 3: several needles
in one point

Needling techniques (see diagram 4):

a) The needle is inserted with a twist, or straight. After one or two minutes it is twisted in a 180 degree motion for 1-2 minutes. This provides a stronger stimulation of the point and is necessary if there is no improvement after 10-15 minutes. (Diagram 4, fig. 1)

b) **Slanted:** The needle is inserted at a 45 or 60 degree angle and then it is either twisted or drawn back and forth under the skin as in a sheath.

c) **One needle for several points** (Diagram 4, fig. 2): The needle can be introduced to a length of 1/2 to 3/4 inch beneath the skin. It is then rotated in 180 degree motions while moving it back and forth at the same time. This can produce very strong reactions and should be stopped as soon as the patient complains of feeling a strong heat in the body, or starts to sweat or feel cold. The needle can then be maintained in place with no further stimulation for 10 minutes.

The advantage of this method is that a whole area of the body can be stimulated since the needle passes through several points at once. For instance, someone may be complaining of pain in the hand, wrist, elbow, shoulder and back. Instead of needling the corresponding points separately, the entire limb can be stimulated at once. In the case of paralysis of a limb, the whole limb can be stimulated with one needle. One is often surprised that after 1 minute or so of this type of stimulation, there can be marked improvement even in motor impairment.

d) **Several needles in one point** (Diagram 4, fig. 3): This method is almost the opposite of the previous one. If one needle is not effective in one point, there will often be an improvement if several needles are placed in the same point. The Chinese have found this method to be more effective than the other methods.

e) **Pecking:** Once the needles are in place on the auricle, a separate needle is used to peck along the helix, without penetrating however. This should not last more than a couple of minutes, after which time the needles that are in place may be twisted several times. Sometimes this can be done before other needles are implanted, so as to prepare the terrain. This procedure

DIAGRAM 5
Electrical treatment for paralysed limbs

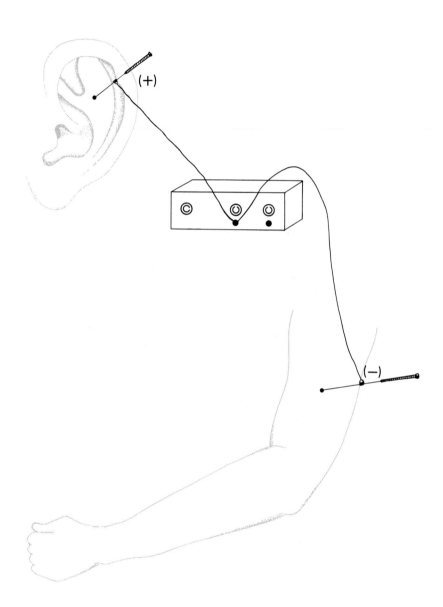

helps to open up the ear meridians that flow internally into the body, allowing the other needles to work more effectively.

f) **Electricity:** An electrical stimulation often produces good results. Apart from the Chinese 71-1 model, there are at the present moment many excellent American and Canadian models available on the market. (It is interesting to note that the Viet-Cong built their own acupuncture stimulators in the midst of the jungle from the electronic equipment of planes that were shot down. The mechanism involved in these machines is simple and can be constructed with parts of an automobile's electronical equipment.)

These machines are useful in that one may attach extra electrodes to them and treat several patients at a time. This comes in handy when treating drug addicts. The only problem is in controlling the wave form, although I believe new machines are being built which allow for connecting different wave forms to different patients at the same time.

If one is using both ears, a positive and a negative electrode are attached to either ear. If only one ear is used, then the negative electrode is placed in the patient's hand and the positive to the ear needle. The intensity of the current is regulated according to the sensation that the patient feels. This should be a slight burning sensation but not pain. There is no danger of the electrode held in the hand causing pain as the intensity of current necessary in the ear is very small.

Electricity is very beneficial in locomotor problems, (Diagram 5) such as involve the use of a limb, for instance. For example in the case of someone suffering from a paralysed arm, the positive electrode is attached to the positive ear arm point or point corresponding to the first dorsal and cervical vertebrae, and the negative electrode placed on the arm of the patient, at a point commanding the muscles and nerves of that limb, such as LI10, 12, or TB10,11. Ear points and body points are combined very beneficially.

g) **Bleeding:** Only one or two drops are bled at each session. This can be done either with a triangular bleeding needle or with a regular needle. It is easiest to obtain blood with a regular needle by inserting the needle and then pulling it out quickly and trying to hook the tip under a part of the skin as it is coming out. This method is useful in high blood pressure. Bleeding one or two points at the back of the ear in the area referred to as the lowering pressure trough, or at the top of the auricle at the Apex point will bring quick relief. The same is true of arteriosclerosis or most blood disorders.

N.B.: Certain people are prone to bleeding. This is especially true of patients suffering from high blood pressure. For this purpose a small cotton ball should be kept close at hand, ready for use, as some people are shocked by the sight of blood. Certain points are situated in areas which have a greater vascularisation and thus tend to bleed more profusely. This is true of the Kidney, Shen Men, and Occiput points. Precautions must be taken to avoid puncturing small superficial blood vessels where these are apparent, unless this is for a specific purpose, such as encouraging better circulation by decongestioning the corresponding body area. The bleeding usually stops after a few seconds, although certain points can bleed longer. The patient may be told to hold onto the cotton ball himself till this dries off.

Type of needle: The thinner the needle the better the reaction. A number 28 needle is generally employed, although a number 30 needle can be used. The needle should be neither too long (over 3/4 inch) nor too heavy so as to avoid unnecessary pain.

h) **Permanent press needles:** These have already been described in the previous pages. They are useful in treating patients who cannot come for treatment as often as necessary, for feeble people, chronic sufferers who react better to a more gradual stimulation, children, and drug addicts (to be described later). The methods of use and the precautions have been described in the section dealing with precautions to take in needling.

i) **Seeds, Ion-spheres:** These have also been described in the previous chapter.

j) **Depth of insertion:** The general rule is that a stronger (Yang) patient needs a deeper penetration than a weak (Yin) patient.

k) **Reaction:** *The type of reaction expressed by the patient determines the curing effect. This is usually expressed as a feeling* *of heat in the auricle, or body, currents flowing through the limbs, or else a temporary aggravation of the symptoms, or a change in the pulse rhythm. Without a reaction there is no curing effect.*

CHAPTER 6

YANG (POSITIVE) REACTIONS

Most ailments cause what is commonly referred to as a "Yang positive reaction" on the auricle. As mentioned before, these reactions appear as discoloration, scars, papules, small tubercles, flaking of skin, purulence, abcesses, exzema, small depressions, etc. The following are some of the general correspondences of Yang reactions to diseases.

Coloration: In Chinese visceral theory, each organ is related to a particular color. Thus:

> Liver & Gall Bladder correspond to Green.
> Heart & Small Intestine correspond to Red.
> Spleen & Stomach correspond to Yellow.
> Lungs & Large Intestine correspond to White.
> Kidneys & Bladder correspond to Black.

For instance, a person whose skin and eyes appear greenish yellow usually has a bad liver. A person whose skin is too pale usually has poor lungs. A skin coloration which is too red is indicative of heart or circulatory problems. Not only can these symptoms be interpreted on the skin of the body and in the eyes, but they appear on the ears as well. Certain ear points, where there is a pathological condition, will have an abnormal coloration compared to the skin immediately surrounding it. According to the precise color of these abnormal spots, we can determine the type of ailment, which other tests will usually confirm, such as lab tests, etc.

Generally speaking we must not forget to begin by looking at the entire ear. An ear whose testure is soft and weak corresponds to a weak constitution. An elastic, supple ear, corresponds to a good physical constitution, with good muscle tone and resistance. A hard ear which will not bend easily, is synonymous to hardened arteries, or calcification of vertebrae and articulations. Thus it is only after having examined the ear in general that one goes on to examine minute details, which will further confirm and point out the exact location of the ailment.

Examination of the entire auricle:

a) **Orange, carroty color:** Spleen disorder, possible polyarthritis, constipation, cholesterol, liver deficiency due to stagnation of blood and "Chi" in the liver, faulty diet.

b) **Pale yellow:** decalcification, arterial and digestive trouble, inefficient spleen, weak stomach, vitamin deficiency, conjunctivitis.

c) **Pale yellow and very dry:** same as above, with possible cancer, ulcers, old chronic condition.

d) **Dark red:** high blood pressure, coronary troubles, hardening of the arteries, low back pain, kidney trouble, loss of memory, violent headaches.

e) **Dark red and hard:** If the cartilage is also hard, this is a sign of very serious vascular trouble with possibility of stroke.

f) **Hard and almost black:** Chronique kidney trouble, near death.

g) **Grayish appearance:** Chronic condition with numerous internal complications, i.e., digestive, circulatory, nervous, etc.

Now we may begin with the small details which appear at particular spots on the auricle.

1) A point which is red or blood shot, whether it be on the rim of the point, whether it appears as a papule, any protuberance, flat red, accompanied by flakiness or not, and having a fatty texture is a symptom of acute and inflammatory condition, localized in the corresponding peripheral area.

2) A white point, flake, papule, depression, swelling, nodule, which is dry and lacking in brightness is indicative of chronic internal trouble.

3) An opaque grey point or swelling may signify a tumor.

4) Husky skin peelings which are difficult to rub off correspond to trouble in absorption such as small intestines, liver, skin, hair.

5) Small scars appear on precise points of the ear after injury by accident or incisions through operations. If there is a red swelling around the scar it may indicate inflammation around the peripheral scar or pain in the scar.

Thus by taking into consideration the above characteristics of color, and texture one may be able to arrive at a fairly accurate diagnosis. This is particularly useful in the country side, or in the case of an emergency when far away from any clinic or hospital. Otherwise it serves to confirm the other findings and sometimes to point out certain disorders that were not obvious upon previous examination.

N.B.: Certain healthy people may present some of these reactions and often one may appear to identify such a reaction whereas in reality there is nothing wrong. If there is no pain felt upon pressing on the point then it is a false reaction, known as a "pseudo-Yang" reaction. Only true painful Yang reactions are considered pathological. Only these will react favorably to needling.

CHINESE VISCERAL THEORY

A knowledge of what each meridian of the body purports to treat will help us to understand the theory behind the selection of certain combinations of points on the ear for the treatment of precise disorders. For instance, why use the Lung point for morphine addiction, or for headache? Why use the Heart point for insomnia or memory?

A) The 3 Yin Hand Meridians

1: Shou Tai Yin (Lungs): The lungs in Chinese medical philosophy are the organs which control the animal instinct, spontaneous reflexes and the skin and hair. Since the meridian passes through the throat and chest and inside of the arm, the lung point on the auricle will control all disorders of these areas. Also there is a secondary branch or meridian which connects it to the head, so that the lung point will prove useful in head-aches localized at the forehead or sinuses.

2: Shou Jue Yin (Heart Constrictor): The heart constrictor, or master of the heart meridian as it is sometimes called, governs pericardium and vascular problems. It is also the controller of sexuality, in that its poor functioning is indicative of either menstrual problems, impotence, or timidity. At the same time the meridian penetrates deeply into the chest and abdomen so that it will be useful in axillar pain, heart conditions, ulcers, and digestive problems.

3: Shou Shao Yin: (Heart): The heart is the ruler of the body in Chinese medicine. It is the king of the castle upon whose good functioning the rest of the castle (body) depends. Also the Chinese place the heart as the center of intelligence and memory. It is the heart that stores the *Shen* or Cosmic principle of Intelligence, and allows it to circulate in the rest of the body. Therefore it is felt that heart problems are moral problems to begin with, problems of expressing one's intelligence. Whereas the master of the heart meridian, and point, treat vascular problems, one must not use the heart point for these. The heart point treats mainly, moral problems, memory, insomnia, pain along the inside of the arm, extending to the auricular finger.

B) The 3 Yang Hand Meridians:

1: Shou Tai Yang (Small Intestine): This is the coupled meridian with the heart. An excess of one usually denotes a lack of energy in the other. Thus the SI point is useful in treating the heart. At the same time it regulates assimilation, moral and physical, so that it can be useful in this type of trouble. The meridian flows upwards along the back of the arm to the scapular region, neck and head and ends in front of the ears. Therefore any trouble in these areas will be treated by the SI point on the auricle. Headaches, at the occiput, deafness, ringing in the ears, eye trouble can all be treated by this point.

2: Shou Shao Yang (Triple Burner): This meridian is coupled with the heart constrictor. These meridians and ear points can be used to regularise each other. The triple burner or San Jiao as it is named in Chinese, is considered one of the most important meridians by many acupuncturists and many treat every disease by this meridian alone. It regulates breathing, digestion, reproductive and eliminatory functions. It is known as the thermo-regulator of the body and is indicated in fevers, glandular deficiencies, sexual problems, nervous disorders, deafness, pain at the temples, and general vitality.

3: Shou Yang Ming (Large Intestine): It is coupled with the lungs and the corresponding auricular point can help to regularize sinus trouble, asthma, bronchitis, nervous disorders. It is also useful to break fevers (by pecking at the LI point for a minute or two). This is the main meridian dealing with dental, facial pain, not to speak of constipation, diarrhea, and hemorrhoids.

We can see from the above that the Yin hand meridians treat mainly the thorax, while the Yang hand meridians are more indicated in treating the head and sense organs.

C) The 3 Yang Foot Meridians:

1: Zu Yang Ming (Stomach): This meridian controls what is referred to as the "Sea Of Nourishment" and sends the Yong nourishing energy circulating in the body. It is also the seat, or the starting point of the triple burners. Since it is coupled with the spleen meridian which is identified with the element earth, the stomach meridian is one of the most important meridians to treat vitality, longevity, physical strength and reasonableness. To speak briefly of the 5-element theory, all other 4 elements must pass through the Earth element which serves to unite them. The Earth element is represented physiologically by the connective tissue. Therefore the stomach point treats not only stomach but also prevents cancer, (if treated at the beginning), and tumors, ulcers, blood trouble, anemia, mouth ulcers, intestinal trouble, and fever.

2: Zu Shao Yang (Gall Bladder): Coupled with the liver, this point on the ear helps to balance the latter. The gall bladder in Chinese visceral theory, is the judge of the body and its function can be compared to a plumb-line in that any imbalance of the body will be reflected by a crispation or looseness of the gall bladder. Thus troubles of equilibrium, dizziness, vertigo, pain at the external corner of the eyes, at the forehead, occiput, ears, throat, chest, ribs, waist, calves, ankles, are treated mainly by the corresponding ear point, mainly on the right ear.

3: Zu Tai Yang (Bladder): This meridian treats pain along its pathway, kidney and bladder trouble, the sexual organs, vitality, headache and fever.

D) The 3 Yin Feet Meridians:

1: Zu Tai Yin (Spleen): The corresponding point treats many of the problems associated with stomach and digestion as well as mouth, and taste, atrophy of limbs, paralysis, reproductive organs, elimination of urine, diabetes, blood deficiencies, mental problems associated with too much thinking.

2 Zu Jue Yin (Liver): The ear point treats mainly reproductive disorders, intestinal and urine elimination as well as lack of vitality, courage, hallucinations such as possession by the devil, spots before the eyes, loss of hair, lack of muscle tone, apathy.

3: Zu Shao Yin (Kidneys): The related point can treat mainly the reproductive organs, urine elimination, excessive fear without cause, will power, ears, hair, heart and lungs.

The 3 Yang foot meridians treat mainly head, sense organs and pain, while the 3 Yin foot meridians treat mainly the abdomen and digestive and reproductive functions.

COMBINING EAR POINTS
WITH BODY POINTS

In many cases it will prove beneficial to combine ear points to body points. This is necessary in many forms of surgery done under acupuncture analgesia. It is also necessary when the ear points alone do not seem to be producing a desirable effect, or vice-versa. One or two body points are usually sufficient to complement the ear points.

To stimulate these body points, one may use the needle alone, or else apply "moxa" to the needle, or electricity, or a moxa cigar or cones. The following is a list of points on the body that are useful in conjunction with auricular points and their chief indications:

1) **Lieh-ch'ueh (Lu 7):** face, nose, forehead, throat.
2) **Chi-zu (Lu 5):** nose, throat, arm, chest, upper back.
3) **Ho-ku (LI 4):** face, teeth, mouth, forehead, chest, sinus, fever.
4) **Shou San-li (LI 10):** arm, vitality, stress, shoulder & back.
5) **Zu San-li (St 36):** front of body, thorax & ribs, digestion, mental disorders, vitality.
6) **San-Yin-jiao (Sp 6):** paralysis, menstrual pain & disorders, stomach, intestines.
7) **Shen-men (He 7):** heart, insomnia, vitality, memory.
8) **Hou-hsi (SI 3):** occiput, head, ears, eyes, neck, back of shoulders, digestion, vitality.
9) **Kao-huang (Bl 43):** anemia, insufficient red blood corpuscles, weak constitution, inability to evacuate phlegm from chest.
10) **Kwun-lun (Bl 60):** sciatica, lumbar pain, mental problems, menstrual trouble.
11) **Cheng-shan (Bl 57):** dorsal view of body, neuro-vegetative reflexes.
12) **Ran-ku (Ki 2):** reproductive system.
13) **Yong-chuan (Ki 1):** paralysis lower limbs, multiple sclerosis.
14) **Nei-kuan (EH 6):** digestion, vitality, vascularisation, fever.

15) **Wai-kuan (TB 5):** deafness, neurasthenia, pain shoulder & back, fever.

16) **Chih-kou (TB 6):** ears, temples, thorax, ribs, skin, intestines.

17) **Kuang-ming (GB 37):** eye trouble.

18) **Xuan-chung (GB 39):** anterior view of body, locomotion, thorax.

19) **Chung-fung (Li 4):** reproductive system.

20) **Chung-kuan (Cv 12):** mid-warmer trouble, stomach ulcers, nerves.

21) **Ming-men (TM 4):** mental and physical vigor, impotence, back pain.

22) **Da-chui (TM 14):** lack of vitality, generalized pain, nerves.

To stimulate any of these points it is preferable to use moxa cigars, though moxa cones (up to 5 in general) or electricity may be employed. The advantage of the cigar is that it maintains a steady heat for a very long time and is less time consuming and less smelly than the other method which consists of placing the moxa directly on the needle. The moxa cigar doesn't have to burn more than a few seconds at a time. Here are a few ways to use this cigar.

1) **For weak or chronic patients,** the burning end of the moxa cigar is held about 1/2 inch away from the point and maintained there until the skin is red at that point. This generally does not take very long and the patient usually complains first that it is too hot. If it is unbearably hot, remove the cigar, rub the skin for a few seconds, and continue until there is a redness. 2-3 applications of this type are usually all that is necessary. One point bilaterally, or on one side, is sufficient in one treatment. It is the initial stimulation which is the most effective, so that it is useless to insist over a longer period of time.

2) **For Yang, stronger patients:** a pecking method is used. The cigar is held above the point and a pecking or flicking motion is exerted with the wrist. The cigar is never put directly in contact with the skin. This can be repeated 4-5 times.

3) the cigar is held above the point and turned in a clockwise motion to supplement a lack of energy, and turned in an anticlockwise motion to disperse an overabundance of energy.

Analysis of Moxa: Analysis of the herb Moxa (from Japanese Mogusa for burning herb), known to us by the Latin name Artemisia Vulgaris, and by the common English name of mugwort reveals the following constituents:

> —Cincol $C_{10}H_{18}O$
> —1 1/2% sesquiterpene
> —1 1/2% sesquiterpene alcohol
> —Artemisin $C_{10}H_{16}N$
> —Adrenin $C_5H_5N_5$
> —Cholin $C_5H_{15}O_2N$
> —Heptaviacontane $C_{31}H_{64}$
> —Tricosanol $C_{23}H_{48}O$
> —Wax
> —Vitamins A, B, C, D.

SECTION III:

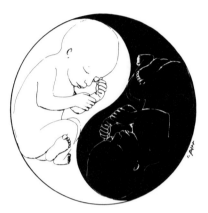

Ear Point Locations
& Treatment

CHAPTER 7

A FEW CASE HISTORIES

In your daily practice, if you are already familiar with acupuncture and are practicing it presently, you come across numerous cases of patients who do not seem to be responding to normal acupuncture treatment. Although you seem to be giving the proper treatment, somehow the patient finds no improvement of his condition. Many factors may be involved, among which the seasonal factor which I have mentioned earlier. Quite often, a patient may respond better in another season. Nevertheless, in such cases, an additional needle or two in the correct ear point will often do the trick, and trigger off the healing mechanism. I can give numerous examples of such cases.

Case I: For example, one female patient of about 56 years of age came to be treated for insomnia. She was addicted to countless drugs that had been prescribed to no avail, and had had psychiatric treatment over a number of years. After 4 treatments with regular acupuncture there was no change. I decided to try a few ear points and inserted two needles, one in the Brain point and one in the Pelvis point. Much to my astonishment, when I came back to see her after 5 minutes, she was fast asleep on the table. I was obliged to wake her up after about an hour. This was the first time in her life since she can recall that she fell asleep so quickly. Although this type of reaction is normal with regular acupuncture, it was the ear points that did it this time. Since then this patient has abandoned all her pills and is an outstanding spokesman for the cause of acupuncture.

Case II: Another interesting case is that of a 74 year old woman suffering from myasthenia facialis. Her mouth would twist involuntarily and her eyes were out of focus in that her peripheral vision remained normal but she saw either nothing at all or else had double vision when looking directly ahead. This time the ear points alone were what was needed. I began the treatment by connecting electrodes to needles implanted in the Mouth and Eye points and providing a slow pulsating current (71-1 Chinese stimulator). This was sufficient to erase the symptoms concerning her mouth and eyes. Each such treatment lasted her approximately 5 days. However, to eradicate the cause itself so that the symptoms should not return at all, I was obliged to stimulate Liver, Lung and Endocrine system points immediately following the other points. After 8 such treatments she no longer presents any grave symptoms and I have her return periodically for a tune-up treatment.

Case III: A man of 62 years of age, was initially suffering from a spasm on the left side of his face which eventually developed into a horrible tic. Normal acupuncture, which is usually very effective in these type of ailments, didn't help at all. I decided to use the ear points. For the first 3 treatments I used 3 needles on the opposite ear and two in the homolateral ear, at the Oesophagus, Stomach, Liver, Cervical Vertebrae, Omega, and Maxillary Articulation points alternately. For the next two treatments I used 2 needles on the opposite ear and three on the corresponding ear, after which only one needle on the opposite ear was necessary for the tic to disappear.

Case IV: One man, 32 years old, who smoked 3 packs of 25 cigarettes a day came to see me for treatment. He smoked 7 cigarettes first thing in the morning before and during his coffee. I was hesitant to treat him and did not promise any results. I used the ears alone, 7 needles in all, 4 in the right ear and 3 in the left. I used the electrical stimulator again for twenty minutes, gradually increasing the pulsations. The points used were the Lung, Palate, Oesophagus, Stomach and Omega points. After the first treatment he couldn't stand the taste of tobacco any longer though his likings for other foods did not change. After 5 treatments he no longer smoked at all. The same sort of reaction was observed with an alcoholic patient though other points were used. The first reaction is a dislike for alcohol.

Case V: A 35 year old man suffering from sciatica. Five normal acupuncture treatments had no effect. An electrical stimulation at the sciatica and lumbar region points erased his pain within 3 treatments at one week intervals and two more treatments at two week intervals.

This type of results are common and are accomplished by many of my colleagues and acupuncturists the world over. The ear point treatment is marvellous at times, and though we may not understand the mechanism of its functioning 100%, it is harmless to try it as the side effects are quite reduced. Moreover the ear points can serve as adjuncts to the body points at times when normal treatment does not give good results. For instance, in certain cases, it may be wise to balance the meridians during one session, and to use the ears on the following one, to pin down the deep rooted problem, or vice-versa. This is extremely effective in the more difficult and dangerous cases, such as inflammatory muscular conditions, multiple sclerosis, diabetes, disc problems, where the needle on the body may actually serve as an irritant and may aggravate the problem. In many cases where pain is the main factor, the ear alone can serve to relieve it literally within seconds.

Case VII: A 48 year old pilot, suffering from rheumatoid arthritis. Cortizone did not help, in that it caused his skin to become extremely fragile and bruise at the slightest touch or pressure. Diet improved his condition somewhat but was not the ultimate solution. This patient was extremely jumpy and wary of needles in his body or limbs, which is quite understandable since here again they may cause grave irritations in the articulations and muscles. It is usually best not to use body points in such cases. The ear points will give results 10 times quicker and without side-effects. The ear points used were those corresponding to the limbs, which were extremely painful on pressure with a probe, and after 5 such treatments, the swelling went down considerably, skin color was almost normal, irritation disappeared for all practical purposes, and use of limbs almost entirely restored. After this initial treatment in 5 sessions, I was able to direct my attention to the emotional, nervous and digestive problems which I suspected were

at the origin of his condition, and my choice of the Dermis, Occiput, Suprarenal, and Triple Burner points proved correct, since
after 4 such treatments he was able to resume his air route without
undue suffering.

Case VIII: A young boy of ten suffering from muscular
dystrophy. His legs were very cramped and his arms too weak to
apply needles. As far as his legs were concerned, I may as well
have put the needles into an iron bar, and as far as his arms were
concerned, I may as well have put the needles into butter. The ear
points gave immediate results. Only two needles were used at the
Cerebellum point. After 2 such treatments he had gained 10% use
of his arms, after two more treatments he gained an additional
10% of his arms. His legs had slightly more mobility, though
nothing spectacular, but the fact that he was able to gain even the
slightest improvement saved both his life and his parent's, who
had tried everything possible without success. At the present he
can walk, though very slowly and awkwardly, but morally he is a
different person.

Case IX: A 53 year old woman, who had her coccyx removed
because of pain in that region and in the rectum. Her tissues were
inflamed and blood vessels apparent and dark blue under a quasi-
transparent skin. After 2 treatments at the Coccyx, Internal
Secretion, Rectum and Dermis points, her complaints were gone.
She returned two months later complaining of a slight tugging at
her rectum. One treatment removed this complaint and has never
returned. Here again, it may have been dangerous to use body
points.

Case X: One woman, 35 years of age, presented herself in our
clinic. She was barely able to walk and appeared in a state of utter
stupor. Upon interrogating her it was found out that she was
taking various tranquilizers and pills for her circulation,
menopause and thyroid. Her voice sounded like a 45 rpm record
turning at 16. She had pain all over her body; it was so ex-
cruciating in her legs that she couldn't wear stockings. Her
memory was a vestige of what it used to be and she had no control
over her balance.

Needless to say the body points would have been of no use
and would only have served to irritate her further. After 4 ear

acupuncture sessions, she was able to wear stockings and the pain only returned 4-5 days after the treatments which were administered at weekly intervals. After 2 more treatments she had cut down her pills to half the quantity she was taking, and after a total of 11 treatments she was only taking one pill for her circulation, which she abandoned after 2 more treatments.

She was given a two month's rest and was readmitted for 3 more sessions after which her condition was judged satisfactory and told to return 6 months later. The complete change that this woman underwent, from a lifeless mummy to a most brilliant and interesting woman was shocking. It seems that the ear points got her out of a depression and daze which had lasted for 12 years.

Case XI; Hollywood, Florida. Upon visiting here I was shocked to find out that one woman, very famous at that, had had her ear removed because of improper use of ear acupuncture. A staple was placed in her ear, such as are now used for the purpose of weight reduction, alcoholism or drug addiction, which is maintained in the ear for several days up to one week. Her ear became infected and had to be cut off.

What happened here is a perfect example of not following the rules for ear acupuncture. Perhaps the infection was due to some other factor of which I am ignorant. Nevertheless, one of the contra-indications of permanent take-home ear needles or staples is warm weather. The weather in Florida is overly warm and humid, a breeding ground for infection! **Permanent ear needles or staples should never be used in very warm and humid weather!** Not observing such elementary precautions is to expose oneself and one's patients to unnecessary trauma. There need be no such occurrences with ear acupuncture. It is impossible to puncture the lungs, or heart or brain, so why not follow a few simple rules such as sterilization, weather conditions and so on and avoid any disasters.

CHAPTER 8

CHINESE EAR POINTS AND THEIR LOCATION*

In the following pages will be found the Chinese ear points and their precise location described anatomically on the ear. The charts on the following pages should be consulted for further verification. I will then go on to present the formulae for combining the points for use in treating pathological conditions. In chapter 10 one will find Nogier's ear points, showing the difference that exists between the two systems and explaining what led to locating the same point at different parts of the ear.

To further simplify the locations of the points on the charts, I have subdivided the ear into anatomical zones, much as the Chinese do, but I have further attributed a different capital letter to each of these zones, so that a person looking up the location of a point on the chart will waste less time in finding it. Thus the letter "A" represents the Lobule, "B" represents the Tragus, . . . as follows: A: Lobule
  B: Tragus
  C: Supra-tragic Incisure
  D: Intertragic Incisure
  E: Antitragus
  F: Antihelix

---

*The numbering here does not correspond to Chinese numbering, as different Chinese works contain different points. I have tried to collect all these points together in a single document.

G: Superior Crus of Antihelix
H: Inferior Crus of Antihelix
I: Triangular Fossa
J: Scapha
K: Helix
L: Crus of Helix
M: Around the Crus of Helix
N: Cymba Conchae
O: Cavum Conchae
P: External Auditory Meatus
Z: Points behind the ear

DIAGRAM 6

Anatomical representation
of body on auricle

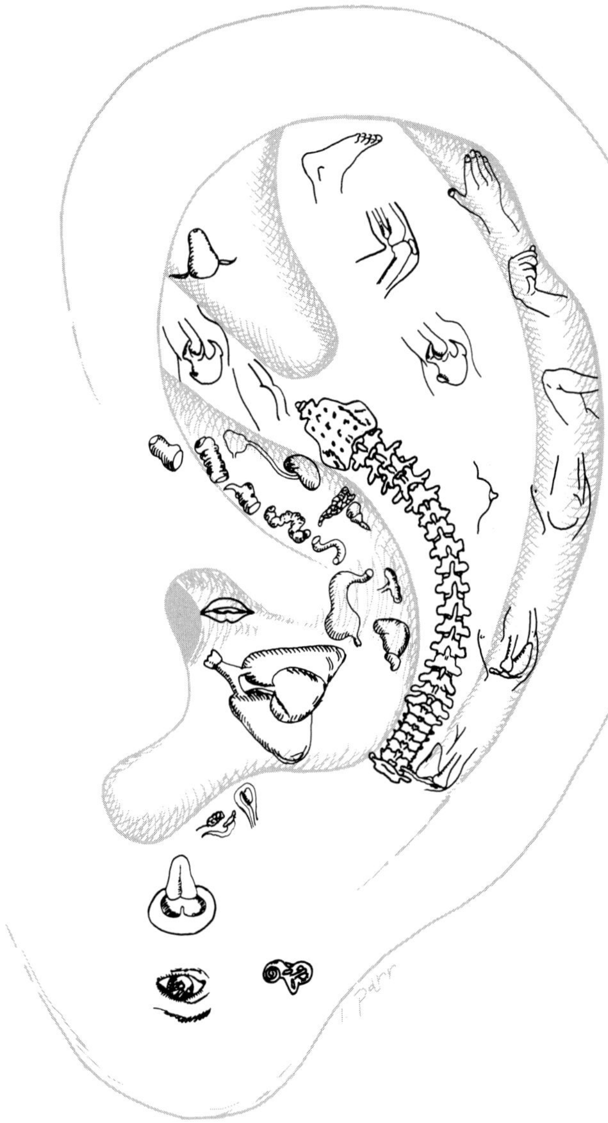

THE POINTS OF THE LOBULE

The points of the lobule are situated in 9 different compartments. The following is the standard division of the lobule into its 9 compartments or areas:

a) Trace a horizontal line (consult diagram 7) immediately at the bottom of the intertragic incisure. This line is divided into three equal parts.

b) Drop two perpendicular lines from each of points dividing the aforementioned horizontal line to the bottom of the lobule.

c) Draw two more lines dividing the ear horizontally in three sections.

d) You now have 9 equal compartments on the lobule. They are numbered from left to right and from top to bottom.

Point	Name of Point	Location
A1	Tooth Extraction Anesthesia point.[1] (upper teeth)	At the postero-inferior part of the first area.
A2	Lower Palate	At the antero-superior part of the second area.
A3	Tongue	At the center of the second area.
A4	Upper Palate	At the postero-inferior part of the second area.
A5	Mandible	Central point of the superior line of the third area.
A6	Tonsil[3]	At the superior border of the third area, where it meets with the middle point of the width of the helix.
A7	Maxilla	The central point of the third area.
A8	Tooth Extraction Anesthesia point[2] (lower teeth)	At the center of the fourth area.
A9	Nervousness point	At the antero-inferior part of the fourth area.

A10	Eye	At the center of the fifth area.
A11	Cheek area	Area around the center of the border between the fifth and sixth areas.
A12	Internal Ear	At the center of the sixth area.
A13	Helix[5]	At the central posterior part of the sixth area, on the rim of the lobule.
A14	Tonsil[4]	At the center of the eighth area.
A15	Helix[6]	At the bottom of the eighth area.
A16	Cancer line	A line following the posterior rim of the lobule, crossing the 3rd, 6th, and up to the middle of 8th area.

THE POINTS ON THE TRAGUS

Point	Name of Point	Location
B1	Apex (nose) of Tragus	The prominent point of the superior projection of the tragus.
B2	Visceral point	Slightly below B1 point, on the free margin of the tragus.
B3	Thirst point	The point at the center of the line connecting B1 and B5.
B4	Pharynx & Larynx	At the inner surface of the tragus, on the opposite side of the external auditory meatus.
B5	External nose	The center point at the bottom of the root of the tragus.
B6	Internal nose	At the inner surface of the tragus, slightly below B4.
B7	Hunger point	The middle point on an imaginary line connecting B5 to B8.
B8	Adrenal gland	The prominent point of the inferior projection of the tragus. If the tragus has a single projection, then this point is immediately below it.

B9   High Blood Pressure   The middle point on the imaginary line connecting point B8 to point Eye[1], in the intertagic incisure.

SUPRA-TRAGIC INCISURE POINTS

Point	Name of Point	Location
C1	External Ear	At the depression in front of the supra-tragic incisure.
C2	Heart point	The mid-point of a line connecting the Apex of Tragus point to the External Ear point, and slightly posterior to it.

INTERTRAGIC INCISURE POINTS

D1	Internal Secretion (Hormone) point.	At the bottom of the incisure.
D2	Ovary	Between the Subcortex point of the antitragus region and the Hormone point (D1).
D3	Eye[1]	At the inferior part of the intertragic incisure and slightly in front of it.
D4	Eye[2]	At the inferior part of the intertragic incisure and slightly behind it.

POINTS OF THE ANTITRAGUS

E1	Brain Axis point	In the middle of the posterior auricular sulcus.
E2	Toothache point	At the inner surface of the point E1 and opposite to E3.

E3	Hou-Ya (Pharynx-tooth)	Between points F1 and E5.
E4	Brain (Pituitary body, Hypophysis)	The central point of the superior third of the brim of the antitragus.
E5	Occiput	At the postero-superior part of the antitragus.
E6	Parotid (salivary) glands	At the center of the middle third of the brim of the antitragus.
E7	Ping-Chuan (Asthma)	At the apex of the antitragus, or at the center of its brim if the apex is not prominent.
E8	Testicle	About 2mm. inside and below the Parotid point (E6) on the medial side of the antitragus.
E9	Forehead	On the cartilage at the inferior third of the external part of the antitragus.
E10	Subcortex (Dermis)	At the inner surface of the antitragus, the central point of the lower third.
E11	Tai Yang (Temples)	The mid-point of the line connecting E5 to E9.
E12	Vertex	About 1.5mm. below Occiput point (E5).

THE POINTS OF THE ANTIHELIX

This region of the ear corresponds to the vertebral column (as shown in diagram 8). Therefore, starting from the posterior auricular sulcus going to the meeting point of the two divisions of the two crurae of the antihelix, the antihelix can be divided from bottom to the top into three parts. The first corresponds to the cervical vertebrae, the second to the thoracic vertebrae and the third to the sacrolumbar vertebrae; the coccyx is located at the point represented by the division of the two crurae.

Point	Name of Point	Location
F1	Cervical vertebrae	Above the posterior auricular sulcus, i.e., at the beginning of the prominent part of the antihelix.
F2	Thoracic vertebrae	In the central part of the antihelix, at the beginning of the 2nd of the 3 divisions of the antihelix.
F3	Lumbosacral vertebrae	At the center of the antihelix, at the beginning of the 3rd area of the antihelix.
F4	Coccygeal vertebrae	At the central point of the end of the antihelix, where it divides into its two roots.
F5	Neck	At the interior border of the antihelix, halfway between F1 and F2.
F6	Thorax	At the interior border of the antihelix, halfway between F2 and F3.
F7	Abdomen	On the interior border of the antihelix, halfway between F3 and F4.
F8	Mammary Gland	Two points on both sides of F2 and above it, with which they form an equilateral triangle.
F9	Thyroid gland	Above point F1, near the scapha.
F10	Outside abdomen	Directly on the opposite side of the antihelix from F7, near the scapha.

POINTS OF THE SUPERIOR CRUS
OF THE ANTIHELIX

G1	Toes	At the postero-superior part of the superior crus.
G2	Heel	At the antero-superior part of the superior crus.
G3	Ankle	Below Heel (G2) and Toe (G1) points together with which it forms an isosceles triangle.

| G4 | Knee | In the center of the superior crus. |
| G5 | Hip | Below and behind the Knee point (G4). |

POINTS OF THE INFERIOR CRUS
OF THE ANTIHELIX

H1	Sympathetic point	On the inferior crus, at the border line where it meets the curved brim of the anterior portion of the helix.
H2	Ischium (sciatic nerve)	Slightly before the middle of the inferior crus.
H3	Buttock	At the inferior part of the margin of the inferior crus.
H4	Lumbago point	Two mm. inside of the Coccyx point (F4).

POINTS OF THE TRIANGULAR FOSSA

I1	Shen Men (Spiritual & Mental Energy point)	Slightly above the meeting point of the two roots of the antihelix, in the triangular fossa.
I2	Pelvic Cavity	Closer to the bifurcation area of the two crurae than point I1.
I3	KuKuan (Coxo-femoral joint).	3mm. above the Ischium (H2) and Buttock (H3) points, with which it forms an equilateral triangle.
I4	Hypotensive point	In the triangular fossa, at the meeting point of the helix with the superior crura.
I5	Uterus	In the triangular fossa, near the helix and halfway between the two crurae.
I6	Asthma (Dyspnea) point	2 mm. below and posterior to the Uterus point (I5).

I7	Hepatitis point	2 mm. behind and slightly above the Uterus point (I5).
I8	Lower section of Rectum	In the triangular fossa, slightly above the Sympathetic point (H1).
I9	Urethra	Halfway between the preceding point (I8) and the Uterus point (I5).
I10	External Genitalia	2mm. above the Uterus (I5) point.

POINTS OF THE SCAPHOID FOSSA

J1	Fingers	Above the level of the auricular (Darwin's) tubercle.
J2	Clavicle	In the scapha, at the same level as a line extended from the Heart point in the concha through the Neck point (F5) on the antihelix.
J3	Shoulder Joint	To localize this point, divide the zone between the Finger point (J1) and Clavicle (J2) into 5 equal compartments. This point is situated in the center of the superior line of the first compartment.
J4	Shoulder	On the superior line of the 2nd compartment, slightly towards the helix.
J5	Elbow	In the center of the superior line of the third compartment.
J6	Wrist	In the middle of the superior line of the 4th compartment.
J7	Appendix[1]	Above the Finger point (J1), towards the superior crus of the antihelix.
J8	Appendix[2]	Beside the Shoulder point (J4), but towards the antihelix.
J9	Appendix[3]	Just below the Clavicle (J2) point.

| J10 | Urticaria Region | Between the Finger (J1) and Wrist (J6) point, bordering on the antihelix. |
| J11 | Minor Occipital Nerve | Above Finger (J1) point and towards the helix. |

THE POINTS OF THE HELIX

K1-6	Helix[1-6]	The 6 Helix points are situated at equal intervals of 6 points beginning from the auricular tubercle downwards to the middle point of the lower margin of the lobule. Helix[6] (K6) is actually situated on, and coincides with point A15; Helix[5] (K5) coincides with lobule point A13.
K7	Tonsil[1]	Draw a perpendicular from Tonsil[4] (A14) to the top of the helix. The meeting point is Tonsil[1].
K8	Tonsil[2]	On the helix, at the summit of an isosceles triangle whose base is formed by the preceding perpendicular.
K9	Tonsil[3]	Same as lobule point A6.
K10	Liver Yang[1]	On the helix, above the auricular tubercle.
K11	Liver Yang[2]	On the helix, below the auricular tubercle.
K12	Apex of Auricle	Fold the ear towards the face. The point is on the pointed part of the helix.
K13	External Genitalia	On the anterior part of the helix, at the same level as the inferior crus of the antihelix.

K14	Urethra	On the anterior portion of the helix, at the same level as the Bladder point in the concha.
K15	Lower Segment of Rectum	On the anterior portion of the helix, at the same level as the Large Intestine point in the concha.
K16	Anus	Between points K14 and K15.
K17	Blind Pile point	On the part of the helix facing the triangular fossa and closer to the superior crura of the antihelix.

POINTS OF THE CRUS OF THE HELIX

| L1 | Diaphragm point | At the lower part of the crus of the helix. |
| L2 | Point of Support | At the end of the crus of the helix, where it meets the concha. |

POINTS AROUND THE CRUS OF THE HELIX

M1	Mouth	Underneath the crus of the helix and above the external auditory meatus.
M2	Oesophagus	Between Mouth point (M1) and Stomach point (M4).
M3	Cardia	Between the preceding point and the Stomach point (M4).
M4	Stomach	In the concha, around the beginning of the crus of the helix.
M5	Duodenum	Above the foot of the crus of the helix and the Stomach point (M4).
M6	Small Intestine	The area immediately following the Duodenum area, just above the crus of the helix.
M7	Appendix	Above the crus of the helix. The area following the Small Intestine area.

M8	Large Intestine	The following area after the Appendix area. It is immediately facing the Mouth area, but on the other side of the crus of the helix.

CYMBA CONCHAE POINTS

N1	Bladder	Above the Large Intestine area point (M8).
N2	Prostate	At the medial side of the preceding point.
N3	Ureter	In between the Bladder (N1) and the Kidney point (N4).
N4	Kidney	Above the Small Intestine point (M6).
N5	Umbilical Region (Drunk Point)	Where the Ureter-Kidney border meets the upper border of the Appendix area.
N6	Pancreas & Gall Bladder	Above the Duodenum (M5) point. The Pancreas is situated on the left ear, whereas on the right ear this area corresponds to the Gall Bladder.
N7	Ascites	Where the Kidney-Pancreas & Gall Bladder border meets the Small Intestine-Duodenum border.
N8	Pancreatitis point	At the lower end of the Pancreas-Gall Bladder border, where it meets the Stomach area.
N9	Liver	Immediately behind the Stomach area, in the postero-inferior part of the cymba concha.
N10	Spleen	The lower half of the Liver on the left auricle. On the right auricle the Liver area belongs exclusively to the liver.

CAVUM CONCHAE POINTS

O1	Heart	The point at the center of the deepest position of the cavum conchae.
O2	Lungs	Lying around the circumference of the Heart point. The area below the Heart corresponds to the Lung on the same side of the body, while the area above the Heart point corresponds to the Lung on the opposite side of the body.
O3	Bronchi	In the Lung region, but towards the external auditory meatus.
O4	Windpipe	Between the Heart point (O1) and the external auditory meatus.
O5	San-Jiao	In between the Internal Nose (B6), Internal Secretion (D1) and Lungs (O2) points.
O6	Muscle relaxing point	On the border between the Spleen and Lungs.

POINTS AROUND THE
EXTERNAL AUDITORY MEATUS

P1	Lower Abdomen	At the superior wall of the external auditory meatus.
P2	Upper Abdomen	At the inferior wall of the external auditory meatus.

POINTS ON THE BACK OF THE AURICLE
(Diagram 9)

The back of the auricle is divided into three zones from top to bottom, representing, the upper back, middle back and lower back respectively. The rim, which is the continuation from the front of the helix, represents the vertebral column and spinal fluid, with the brain at the top and the perineum at the lower end.

Point	Name of Point	Location
Z1	Bleeding & Depressing Groove	The superior third of the curved verticle groove at the back of the auricle.
Z2	Upper Back	Above the upper cartilaginous eminence.
Z3	Middle Back	Along the middle of the back of the auricle.
Z4	Lower Back	Below the cartilaginous eminence.
Z5	Top of Brain	At the top of the back of the auricle.
Z6	Spinal cord[1]	Just inside of the preceding point, near the Depressing groove (Z1).
Z7	Antipyretics	On the back of the helix, at the level of the upper back delineation.
Z8	Tin Ying	4 mm. below above point.
Z9	Headache[1]	Just below the Upper Back section, close to the verticle ridge separating the ear from the mastoid process.
Z10	Headache[2]	4 mm. below and more inward than the preceding point.
Z1	Headache[3]	At approximately the same level as the above point, 1 mm. higher, and closer to the Hypotensive (Depressing) groove.
Z12	Neck	About. 4 mm. below and slightly more inward than Headache[2] (Z10).
Z13	Sedation	At the level of the cartilaginous eminence at the back of the auricle, close to the mastoid, slightly above it and exterior to it.
Z14	Brain Chi	At a level halfway between the preceding two points but more outward.
Z15	Groove[1]	Below the preceding point, about 4mm.

Z16	Groove²	Just above the Middle Back delineation, close to the groove formed by the back of the antihelix.
Z17	Epigastric Region	At the same level as the preceding point but more inward, towards the mastoid.
Z18	Nerve Center	A few mm. below and slightly more inward than the Tin Ying point (Z8).
Z19	Vertebral Column	Halfway between the preceding point and Backache¹ point (Z20).
Z20	Backache¹	Halfway between the preceding point and Backache² more inward, close to the downward extension of the Depressing Groove.
Z21	Backache²	On the back of the antihelix part of the auricle, at the level of the Middle Back.
Z22	Fauces	Just below the Middle Back area line, at the halfway mark.
Z23	Groove³	At about the same level as the preceding point, but close to the extension of the Depressing Groove.
Z24	Ulcer	Halfway between the two preceding points, but below them, forming an equilateral triangle with them.
Z25	Back	Below Backache² point (Z21), same distance below it as Backache¹ (Z20) is above it.
Z26	Lung	Same distance below preceding point as the preceding point is from the one above (Z21). Closer to the Hypotensive (Depressing) Groove.
Z27	Lumbago	About 2mm. below and exterior to the preceding point.
Z28	Mesogastric Region	About 2mm. below the preceding

		point, but close to the extension of the Depressing Groove.
Z29	Cough & Asthma	2-3mm. behind and slightly below the preceding point.
Z30	Hypogastric Region	The summit point of an isosceles triangle formed with the above point and the one below (Z31).
Z31	Buttock	In the middle of the area corresponding to the back of the antihelix, at the level of the Lower Back line.
Z32	Gastro-Intestinal Tract	Halfway between the Middle Back and Lower Back lines, but only a few mm. from the groove separating the auricle from the mastoid.
Z33	Epigastric Region	At the same level as the preceding point, but close to the back of the antihelix.
Z36	Heart	Behind the Heart point in the front of the auricle, in the concha. Slightly below and about halfway between the two preceding points.
Z35	Kidney Cell	2.5mm. below point Z32 (Gastro-Intestinal Tract).
Z36	Pai Ling	2.5mm. below the above point.
Z37	Yang Ho	2.5mm. below the above point, just above the Lower Back line.
Z38	Appendix	At the same level as Pai Ling (Z36), close to the back of the antihelix.
Z39	Pai Ling	At the same verticle level as the above point, but just below the Lower Back line.
Z40	Lower Extremities	Below the Lower Back line, about 5mm. below Yang Ho point (Z37).
Z41	Ear	At the bottom of the back of the auricle, close to where the auditory canal is felt.

Z42	Perineum[1]	Halfway between Pai Ling (Z39) and Yi Shan (Z43).
Z43	Yi Shan	In back of the area corresponding to the top of the antitragus, where the lobule joins with the cartilage at the back of the auricle.
Z44	Perineum[2]	On the area corresponding to the back of the helix and antihelix, forming with the above two points an equilateral triangle.
Z45	Spinal Cord[2]	On the back of the concha: the summit of an isosceles triangle formed with the points Perineum[1] (Z42) and Yi Shan (Z43).
Z46	Yi Len	Below Yi Shan (Z43), at the bottom of the back of the lobule.

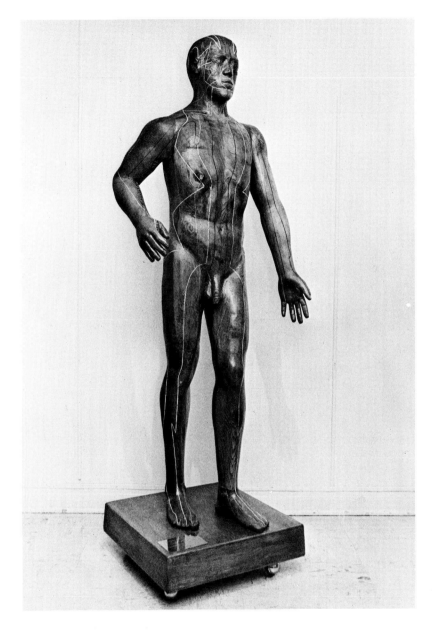

"L'Homme du Quebéc," a life-size acupuncture statue used by students to locate the points and practice needling.

Sculpture: Jacques Edward Bourque

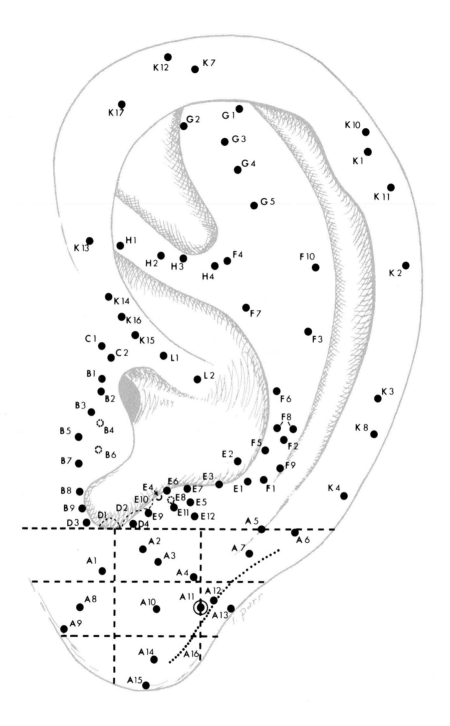

DIAGRAM 7
Points on the outward portions of the auricle

A1	Tooth Extraction Anesthesia point-[1] (upper teeth)	E8	Testicle
A2	Lower Palate	E9	Forehead
A3	Tongue	E10	Subcortex (Dermis)
A4	Upper Palate	E11	Tai Yang (Temples)
A5	Mandible	E12	Vertex
A6	Tonsil[3]	F1	Cervical Vertebrae
A7	Maxilla	F2	Thoracic Vertebrae
A8	Tooth Extraction Anesthesia point-[2] (lower teeth)	F3	Lumbosacral Vertebrae
		F4	Coccygeal Vertebrae
A9	Nervousness point		
A10	Eye	F5	Neck
A11	Cheek area	F6	Thorax
A12	Internal Ear	F7	Abdomen
A13	Helix[5]	F8	Mammary Gland
A14	Tonsil[4]	F9	Thyroid Gland
A15	Helix[6]	F10	Outside Abdomen
A16	Cancer line	G1	Toes
B1	Apex of Tragus	G2	Heel
B2	Visceral point	G3	Ankle
B3	Thirst point	G4	Knee
B4	Pharynx & Larynx	G5	Hip
B5	External Nose	H1	Sympathetic point
B6	Internal Nose	H2	Ischium (Sciatic Nerve)
B7	Hunger point	H3	Buttock
B8	Adrenal Gland	H4	Lumbago point
B9	High Blood Pressure	K1	Helix[1]
C1	External Ear	K2	Helix[2]
C2	Heart point	K3	Helix[3]
D1	Internal Secretion (Hormone) point	K4	Helix[4]
		K7	Tonsil[1]
D2	Ovary	K8	Tonsil[2]
D3	Eye[1]	K9	Tonsil[3]
D4	Eye[2]	K10	Liver Yang[1]
E1	Brain Axis point	K11	Liver Yang[2]
E2	Toothache point	K12	Apex of the Auricle
E3	Hou-Ya (Pharynx-tooth)	K13	External Genitalia
E4	Brain (Pituitary body, Hypophysis)	K14	Urethra
		K15	Lower Segment of Rectum
E5	Occiput	K16	Anus
E6	Parotid glands	K17	Blind Pile point
E7	Ping-Chuan (Asthma)	L1	Diaphragm point
		L2	Point of Support

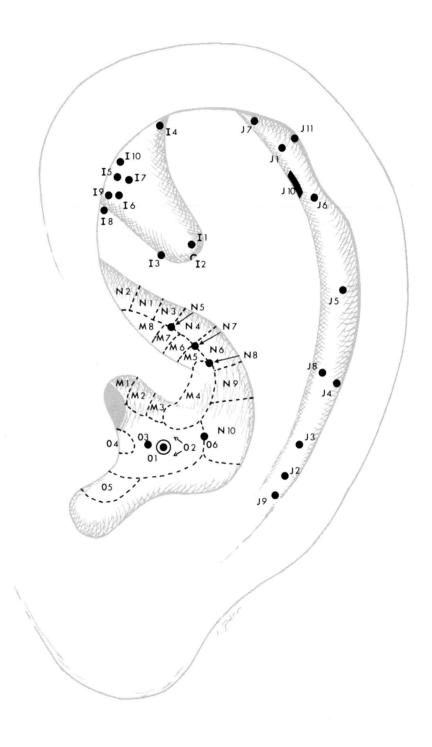

DIAGRAM 8
Points appearing in the concave portions
of the anterior surface of the auricle

I1 Shen Men (Spiritual & Mental Energy point)
I2 Pelvic Cavity
I3 Ku-Kuan (Coxo-femoral joint)
I4 Hypotensive point
I5 Uterus
I6 Asthma (Dyspnea) point
I7 Hepatitis point
I8 Lower Section of Rectum
I9 Urethra
I10 External Genitalia
J1 Fingers
J2 Clavicle
J3 Shoulder Joint
J4 Shoulder
J5 Elbow
J6 Wrist
J7 Appendix[1]
J8 Appendix[2]
J9 Appendix[3]
J10 Urticaria Region
J11 Minor Occipital Nerve
M1 Mouth
M2 Oesophagus
M3 Cardia
M4 Stomach
M5 Duodenum
M6 Small Intestine
M7 Appendix
M8 Large Intestine
N1 Bladder
N2 Prostate
N3 Ureter
N4 Kidney
N5 Umbilical Region (Drunk point)
N6 Pancreas & Gall Bladder
N7 Ascitis
N8 Pancreatitis point
N9 Liver
N10 Spleen

O1 Heart
O2 Lungs
O3 Bronchi
O4 Windpipe
O5 San-Jiao (Chiao)
O6 Muscle Relaxing Point
P1 Lower Abdomen
P2 Upper Abdomen

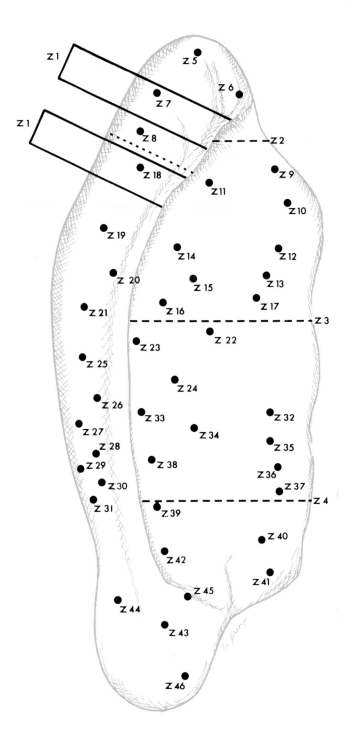

DIAGRAM 9
Points on the posterior auricle

Z1 Bleeding & Hypotensive
    Groove
Z2 Upper Back
Z3 Middle Back
Z4 Lower Back
Z5 Top of Brain
Z6 Spinal Cord[1]
Z7 Antipyretics
Z8 Tin Ying
Z9 Headache[1]
Z10 Headache[2]
Z11 Headache[3]
Z12 Neck
Z13 Sedation
Z14 Brain Chi
Z15 Groove[1]
Z16 Groove[2]
Z17 Epigastric Region
Z18 Nerve Center
Z19 Vertebral Column
Z20 Backache[1]
Z21 Backache[2]
Z22 Fauces
Z23 Groove[3]
Z24 Ulcer
Z25 Back
Z26 Lung
Z27 Lumbago
Z28 Mesogastric Region
Z29 Cough & Asthma
Z30 Hypogastric Region
Z31 Buttock
Z32 Gastro-Intestinal Tract
Z33 Epigastric Region
Z34 Heart
Z35 Kidney Cell
Z36 Pai Ling
Z37 Yang Ho
Z38 Appendix
Z39 Pai Ling
Z40 Lower Extremities
Z41 Ear
Z42 Perineum[1]

Z43 Yi Shan
Z44 Perineum[2]
Z45 Spinal Cord[2]
Z46 Yi Len

CHAPTER **9**

EAR ACUPUNCTURE TREATMENT

EAR ACUPUNCTURE TREATMENTS

SUBJECT: INTERNAL MEDICINE

DISEASES	MAJOR POINTS	SECONDARY POINTS
Infectious diseases		
Common Cold	Internal Nose-B6, Adrenal Gland-B8, Forehead-E9, Lung-02.	Subcortex (Dermis)-E10; Occiput-E5.
Varicella	Lung-O2; Internal Secretion-D1; Adrenal Gland-B8; Occiput-E5; Shen Men-I1.	
Epidemic Parotitis	Parotid gland-E6; Internal Secretion-D1; Cheeks-A11; Dermis-E10.	
Acute & Chronic Infectious Hepatitis	Liver-N9; Sympathetic-H1; Shen Men-I1; Spleen-N10.	Liver-Yang^1 & $^{-2}$-K10 & K11; Gall Bladder-N6; Internal Secretion-D1; Kidney-N4.
Pertussis (100 Day Cough)	Lung-O2; Bronchi;O3; Adrenal Gland-B8; Shen Men-I1; Ping Chuan-E7.	Sympathetic-H1; Occiput-E5.
Bacterial Dysentery	Large Intestine-M8; Small Intestine-M6; Lower Segment of Rectum-K15; Shen Men-I1; Internal Secretion-D1; Occiput-E5; Lung-O2; Sympathetic-H1.	

	Condition	Treatment Points	
Infectious Diseases	Phthisis	Lung-O2; Thorax-F6; Adrenal Gland-B8; Internal Secretion-D1.	Subcortex (Dermis)-E10; San Jiao-O5.
	Malaria	Subcortex (Dermis)-E10; Internal Secretion-D1; Liver-N9; Spleen-N10; Adrenal Gland-B8.	
Diseases of the Digestive System	Acute & Chronic Gastritis	Stomach-M4; Sympathetic-H1; Shen Men-I1; Spleen-N10; Lung-O2.	Abdomen-F7.
	Gastric Ulcer	Same as above.	Subcortex-E10; Duodenum-M5.
	Duodenal Ulcer	Duodenum-M5; Sympathetic-H1; Shen Men-I1.	Subcortex-E10; Stomach-M4; Lung-O2.
	Gastroptosis	Stomach-M4; Sympathetic-H1; Subcortex (Dermis)-E10.	Shen Men-I1; Liver-N9.
	Spasm of the Stomach	Stomach-M4; Liver-N9; Sympathetic-H1; Shen Men-I1.	Upper Abdomen-P2; Lower Abdomen-P1.
	Gastro-enteric Neurosis	Same as above.	Duodenum-M5.
	Musculophrenic Spasm	Diaphragm-L1; Shen Men-I1; Subcortex-E10; Ear Apex-K12.	
	Enteritis	Large Intestine-M8; Lower segment of Rectum-K15; Sympathetic-H1; Shen Men-I1.	Small Intestine-M6; Spleen-N10.
	Eructation	Shen Men-I1; Stomach-M4; Sympathetic-H1.	Windpipe-O4.
	Anaphylactic Colitis	Large Intestine-M8; Internal Secretion-D1; Sympathetic-H1; Lungs-O2.	Shen Men-I1; Small Intestine-M6.

Condition	Prescription	
Appendix Pain	Appendix-M7; Shen Men-I1; Sympathetic-H1.	Stomach-M4; Subcortex (Dermis)-E10.
Intestinal Tuberculosis	Large Intestine-M8; Small Intestine-M6; Sympathetic-H1; Shen Men-I1; Internal Secretion-D1.	Occiput-E5; San Jiao-O5.
Indigestion	Small Intestine-M6; Sympathetic-H1; Stomach-M4; Pancreas-Gall Bladder-N6; Spleen-N10.	Large Intestine-M8; San Jiao-O5; Shen Men-I1.
Nausea & Vomiting	Stomach-M4; Shen Men-I1; Occiput-E5; Sympathetic-H1.	Subcortex (Dermis)-E10; Oesophagus-M2.
Diarrhea	Large Intestine-M8; Small Intesting-M6; Sympathetic-H1; Shen Men-I1.	Lower segment of the Rectum-K15; Spleen-N10.
Constipation	Large Intestine-M8; Lower segment of Rectum-K15; Subcortex (Dermis)-E10.	Sympathetic-H1; Spleen-N10.
Distended abdomen	Small Intestine-M6; Large Intestine-M8; Stomach-M4; Sympathetic-H1.	Abdomen-F7; San Jiao-O5.
Intestinal Colic	Small Intestine-M6; Sympathetic-H1; Shen Men-I1; Ear Apex-K12.	Upper Abdomen-P2; Lower Abdomen-P1.
Functional Disturbances of the Stomach & Intestine	Stomach-M4; Small Intestines-M6; Large Intestine-M8; Sympathetic-H1.	Shen Men-I1; Spleen-N10; San Jiao-O5.
Cholecystitis	Sympathetic-H1; Shen Men-I1; Gall Bladder-N6; Liver-N9.	Adrenal Gland-B8.

Cholepyrrhin	Same as above.	Subcortex-E10; Muscle relaxing point-O6.
Gall Bladder (parasites)	Same as above.	Subcortex (Dermis)-E10.
Diseases of the Respiratory System		
Bronchitis	Bronchi-O3; Shen Men-I1; Ping Chuan-E7; Adrenal Gland-B8.	Sympathetic-H1; Occiput-E5.
Tracheitis	Windpipe-O4; Same as above except Bronchi.	Same as above.
Lobar Pneumonia	Lung-O2; Thorax-F6; Adrenal Gland-B8; Internal Secretion-D1.	Shen Men-I1; Subcortex-E10.
Broncho-Pneumonia	Lung-O2; Bronchi-O3; Sympathetic-H1; Shen Men-I1; Ping Chuan-E7.	Adrenal Galnd-B8; Occiput-E5; Internal Secretion-D1.
Asthma	Sympathetic-H1; Shen Men-I1; Ping Chuan-E7; Adrenal Gland-B8.	Lung-O2; Occiput-E5; Internal Secretion-D1.
Alveolar Emphysema	Lung-O2; Bronchi-O3; Sympathetic-H1; Shen Men-I1; Ping Chuan-E7.	Occiput-E5; Adrenal Gland-B8.
Shortness of Breath	Inner Nose-B6; Adrenal Gland-B8; Forehead-E9; Shen Men-I1.	Lung-Z25.
Pleurisy	Lung-O2; Thorax-F6; Adrenal Gland-B8; Internal Secretion-D1.	Subcortex-E10; San Jiao-O5.
Pleural Adhesions	Thorax-F6; Adrenal Gland-B8; Internal Secretion-D1.	Subcortex-E10; Shen Men-I1.

Cough (recent)	Ping Chuan-E7; Shen Men-I1; Lung-O2.	Occiput-E5; Windpipe-O4; Adrenal Gland-B8.
Cough (chronic)	Shen Men-I1; Ping Chuan-E7; Windpipe-O4; Lung-O2; Sympathetic-H1.	Occiput-E5; Adrenal Gland-B8.
Pressure on Chest	Sympathetic-H1; Heart-O1; Thorax-F6.	Occiput-E5; Lung-O2.
Chest Pain	Shen Men-I1; Heart-O1; Sympathetic-H1; and related points to the locality.	Stomach-M4; Subcortex-E10.
Diseases of the Circulatory System — Myocarditis	Heart-O1; Small Intestine-M6; Sympathetic-H1; Shen Men-I1.	Occiput-E5.
Rheumatoid Cardiopathy	Heart-O1; Internal secretion-D1; Sympathetic-H1; Shen Men-I1.	Small Intestion-M6; Subcortex-E10.
High Blood Pressure	Depressing Point-I4; Hypotensive Groove-Z1; (blood-letting); Sympathetic-H1; Shen Men-I1; Heart-O1.	
Cardiac Arrhythmia	Heart-O1; Sympathetic-H1; Shen Men-I1.	Subcortex-E10.
Low Blood Pressure	Sympathetic-H1; Heart-O1; Occiput-E5; Adrenal Gland-B8.	
Buerger's Disease	Sympathetic-H1; Kidney-N4; Heart-O1; Adrenal Gland-B8; Liver-N9; Spleen-N10.	Internal Secretion-D1; Subcortex-E10; Occiput-E5.
Inflammation of Arterial Wall	Sympathetic-H1; Kidney-N4; Heart-O1; Adrenal Gland-B8; Liver-N9.	Spleen-N10; Occiput-E5; Internal Secretion-D1.

	Peripheral Circulatory Disturbances	Corresponding regions; Internal Secretion-D1; Adrenal Gland-B8.	
	Coronary Thrombosis	Heart-O1; Sympathetic-H1; Internal Secretion-D1; Adrenal Gland-B8.	Small Intestine-M6; Kidney-N4; Subcortex-E10.
Diseases of the Blood System	Hypoferric Anemia	Liver-N9; Spleen-N10; Internal Secretion-D1; Diaphragm-L1.	Stomach-M4; Small Intestine-M6.
	Leukopenia	Liver-N9; Spleen-N10; Heart-O1; Kidney-N4; Internal Secretion-D1.	Occiput-E5; Diaphragm-L1; Smypathetic-H1.
	Thrombopenic Purpura	Liver-N9; Spleen-N10; Diaphragm-L1; Sympathetic-H1; Shen Men-I1; Internal Secretion-D1.	Occiput-E5; Heart-O1.
Diseases of the Urinary and Generative System	Acute Nephritis	Kidney-N4; Urinary Bladder-N1; Sympathetic-H1; Shen Men-I1; Liver-N9.	Adrenal Gland-B8; Internal Secretion-D1.
	Nephropathic Syndrome	Kidney-N4; Urinary Bladder-N1; Sympathetic-H1; Shen Men-I1; Ascites-N7.	Adrenal Gland-B8.
	Pyelonephritis	Kidney-N4; Urinary Bladder-N1; Sympathetic-H1; Shen Men-I1; Liver-N9..	Adrenal Gland-B8; Internal Secretion-D1.
	Diminution of Kidney Function	Kidney-N4; Urinary Bladder-N1; Sympathetic-H1; Shen Men-I1.	Adrenal Gland-B8; Occiput-E5.
	Hematuria	Kidney-N4; Urinary Bladder-N1; Liver-N9; Diaphragm-L1; Adrenal gland-B8.	
	Pollakiuria; Precipitant Urination	Urinary Bladder-N1; Kidney-N4; Shen Men-I1.	

	Condition	Points
	Retention of Urine	Kidney-N4; Urinary Bladder-N1; Sympathetic-H1; External Genital Organs-K13. Subcortex-E10.
	Incontinence of Urine	Urinary Bladder-N1; Brain-E4; Point of Support-L2.
	Impotence	Uterus-I5; External Genitalia-K13; Testicle-E8; Internal Secretion-D1; Kidney-N4.
	Ejaculatio Praecox	Uterus-I5; External Genitalia-K13; Testicle-E8; Internal Secretion-D1; Shen Men-I1.
	Cystitis	Urinary Bladder-N1; Kidney-N4; Sympathetic-H1; Occiput-E5; Adrenal gland-B8.
	Urinary Lithiasis	Ureter-N3; Kidney-N4; Sympathetic-H1; Subcortex-E10; Urinary Bladder-N1.
	Orchitis	Testicle-E8; Internal Secretion-D1; Shen Men-I1; Adrenal Gland-B8. External Genitalia-K13.
	Epididymitis	Same as above. Same, plus Ku-Kuan-I3.
	Prostatitis	Prostate-N2; Urinary Bladder-N1; Internal Secretion-D1; Kidney-N4. Occiput-E5.
Disease of the Endocrine System	Hypophysial Dwarfism	Kidney-N4; Internal Secretion-D1; Brain-E4. Testicle-E8 (male); Ovary-D2 (female).
	Hypothyroidism	Thyroid-F9; Internal Secretion-D1; Brain-E4; Shen Men-I1.
	Hyperthyroidism	Same as above. Cervical Vertebrae-F1.

	Sheehan's Disease	Brain-E4; Liver-N9; Spleen-N10; Sympathetic-H1; Uterus-I5; Internal Secretion-D1.	
	Diabetes Insipidus	Brain-E4; Internal Secretion-D1; Sympathetic-H1; Shen Men-I1; Kidney-N4; Bladder-N1.	
	Secretory Disturbances	Internal Secretion-D1; Brain-E4; Subcortex-E10; Spleen-N10.	Testicle-E8 (male); Ovary-D2 (female).
	Gynecomastia	Internal Secretion-D1; Brain-E4; Mammary gland-F8.	
Diseases of the Locomotor System	Torticollis	Cervical Vertebrae-F1; Neck-F5; Shen Men-I1.	
	Hypertrophic Spondylopathy	Points corresponding to the region; Internal Secretion-D1; Adrenal Gland-B8; Subcortex-E10.	Kidney-N4; Shen Men-I1.
	Periarthritis of the Shoulder	Shoulder Joing-J3; Shoulder-J4; Shen Men-I1.	Clavicle-J2; Adrenal gland-B8.
	Rheumatoid Arthritis	Shen Men-I1; Kidney-N4; Internal Secretion-D1; Occiput-E5; corresponding points.	Subcortex-E10.
	Joint Friction	Corresponding points to the region; Internal secretion-D1; Adrenal Gland-B8; Subcortex-E10.	Kidney-N4; Shen Men-I1.
	Osteomalacia of the Patella	Corresponding points to the region; Internal secretion-D1; plus same as above.	Same as above.
Diseases of the Mental and Nervous System	Trigeminal Neuralgia	Cheeks-A11; Upper Jaw-A7; Lower Jaw-A5; Shen Men-I1; Occiput-E5.	External Ear-C1.
	Facial Nerve Paralysis	Cheeks-A11; Occiput-E5; Eye-A10; Mouth-M1.	Upper Jaw-A7; Lower Jaw-A5; Liver-N9.

Facial Spasms	Cheeks-A11; Shen Men-I1; Subcortex-E10; Tai Yang-E11.	Subcortex-E10; Stomach-M4.
Meuniere's Disease	Kidney-N4; Shen Men-I1; Occiput-E5; Internal Ear-A12.	Adrenal Gland-B8.
Intercostal Neuralgia	Thorax-F6; Occiput-E5.	
Ischialgia	Ischium-H2; Shen Men-I1; Kidney-N4; Occiput-E5.	
Multiple Neuritis	Points corresponding to the region; Shen Men-I1; Adrenal Gland-B8; Internal Secretion-D1.	
Amyotrophic Lateral Sclerosis	Kidney-N4; Internal Secretion-D1; Brain Axis-E1; Occiput-E5; San Jiao-O5.	Kidney-N4; Shen Men-I1.
Cerebellar Ataxia	Brain Axis-E1; Occiput-E5; Cervical Vertebrae-F1	Subcortex-E10.
Epilepsy	Shen Men-I1; Kidney-N4; Occiput-E5; Heart-O1; Stomach-M4.	Stomach-M4; Subcortex-E10.
Sequela of Commotio Cerebri	Kidney-N4; Brain Axis-E1; Occiput-E5; Shen Men-I1; Heart-O1.	Stomach-M4; Subcortex-E10.
Sequela of Cerebral Meningitis	Same as above.	Same as above.
Sequela of Infantile Paralysis	Corresponding to the region; Shen Men-I1; Adrenal gland-B8; Internal Secretion-D1.	Subcortex-E10; Occiput-E5.

Diseases of the Mental and Nervous System		
Sequela of Cerebral Hemorrhage	Corresponding to the region; Shen Men-I1; Adrenal gland-B8; Internal Secretion-D1.	Subcortex-E10; Occiput-E5.
Sequela of Polio	Corresponding to the region; same as above.	Same as above.
Atelencephalia	Kidney-N4; Occiput-E5; Brain Axis-E1; Shen Men-I1; Subcortex-E10.	Internal Secretion-D1; Forehead-E9.
Migraine	Tai Yang-E11; Shen Men-I1; Kidney-N4; Subcortex-E10.	
Hyperhydrosis	Sympathetic-H1; Lung-O2; Internal Secretion-D1; Occiput-E5; Adrenal Gland-B8.	
Headache; Dizziness	Occiput-E5; Forehead-E9; Shen Men-I1; Subcortex-E10.	
Insomnia; frequent dreams	Shen Men-I1; Heart-O1; Kidney-N4; Occiput-E5.	
Neurasthenia	Heart-O1; Kidney-N4; Shen Men-I1; Occiput-E5; Stomach-M4.	Subcortex-E10.
Hysteria (and loss of memory)	Heart-O1; same as above and, Brain Axis-E1.	Same as above.
Hysteric Aphasia	Brain-E4; Occiput-E5; Heart-O1; Shen Men-I1; Kidney-N4; Subcortex-E10.	
Hysteric Paralysis	Subcortex-E10; Shen Men-I1; Occiput-E5; Heart-O1; corresponding area.	Stomach-M4; Kidney-N4.

Schizophrenia	Kidney-N4; Shen Men-I1; Occiput-E5; Heart-O1; Stomach-M4; Brain Axis-E1. Subcortex-E10.
Hallucination	Kidney-N4; Liver-N9; Eye-A10; Occiput-E5.
Shock	Adrenal Gland-B8; Occiput-E5; Heart-O1; Brain-E4; Subcortex-E10.
Excessive Sweating	Sympathetic-H1; Lung-O2; Internal Secretion-D1; Occiput-E5; Adrenal gland-B8.
Alcoholism	Lower Segment of Rectum-K15; Diaphragm-L1; Point of Support-L2.
Tobacco Addiction	Lower Jaw-A5; Upper Jaw-A7; Tongue-A3.
Drug Addiction	Lung-O2; Liver-N9; Kidney-N4; Shen Men-I1; Adrenal Gland-B8. Brain Axis-E1; Subcortex-E10; Occiput-E5.

SUBJECT: SURGERY

DISEASES	MAJOR POINTS	SECONDARY POINTS
Furuncle, Carbuncle and Paronychia	Corresponding area; Shen Men-I1; Occiput-E5; Adrenal Gland-B8.	
Cellulitis	Corresponding area; Adrenal Gland-B8; Shen Men-I1; Spleen-N10.	
Erysipelas	Corresponding area (pecking): Lung-O2; Occiput-E5; Adrenal Gland-B8; Internal Secretion-D1; Shen Men-I1.	
Mastitis	Mammary Gland-F8; Internal Secretion-D1; Occiput-E5; Adrenal Gland-E5; Thorax-F6.	
Mammary Abscess	Same as above.	
Acute and Chronic Appendicitis	Appendix-M7; Large Intestine-M8; Sympathetic-H1; Shen Men-I1; Lung-O2.	Liver-N9; Duodenum-M5.
Cholelithiasis	Gall Bladder-N6; Sympathetic-H1; Shen Men-I1.	
Round-Worms in Biliary Tract	Same as above.	Same as above.
Chronic Cholecystitis	Gall Bladder-N6; Liver-N9; Sympathetic-H1; Shen Men-I1.	Internal Secretion-D1.
Chronic Pancreatitis	Pancreas-N6; Internal Secretion-D1; Sympathetic-H1; Shen Men-I1.	

Paralytic Intestinal Obstruction	Large Intestine-M8; Small Intestine-M6; Sympathetic-H1; Subcortex-E10; Abdomen-F7.	
Renal Calculus	Kidney-N4; Ureter-N3; Sympathetic-H1; Shen Men-I1;	Subcortex-E10.
Uresteral Calculus	Ureter-N3; Kidney-N4; Sympathetic-H1; Shen Men-I1.	
Incomplete Hernia	Lower Abdomen-P1; Subcortex-E10; Internal Secretion-D1.	
Anal Fissure	Lower Segment of Rectum-K15; Shen Men-I1.	Large Intestine-M8; Spleen-N10; Lung-O2.
Prolapse of Anus	Lower Segment of Rectum-K15; Large Intestine-M8; Subcortex-E10.	Spleen-N10.
Internal Piles; External Piles	Lower segment of rectum-K15; Large Intestine-M8.	Subcortex-E10; Spleen-N10; Adrenal Gland B8.
Cystitis	Urinary Bladder-N1; Kidney-N4; Sympathetic-H1; Shen Men-I1.	Occiput-E5; Adrenal Gland B8.
Prostatitis	Prostate-N2; Urinary Bladder-N1; Internal Secretion-D1; Kidney-N4.	Occiput-E5.
Orchitis; Epididymitis	Testicle-E8; Internal Secretion-D1; Shen Men-I1; Adrenal gland-B8.	External Genitalia-I10; Ku-Kuan-I3.
Habitual Dislocation of Joint	Corresponding area; Internal Secretion-D1; Adrenal Gland-B8; Subcortex-E10; Spleen-N10; Liver-N9.	
Fracture, Contusion, Sprain and Crushed Injury	Corresponding to the region; Shen Men-I1; Kidney-N4; Subcortex-E10.	Adrenal gland-B8.

Bone Spicula after Arthritis or Periostitis	Kidney-N4; Internal Secretion-D1; Occiput-E5; Adrenal Gland-B8; corresponding to area.	

SUBJECT: GYNECOLOGY

DISEASES	MAJOR POINTS	SECONDARY POINTS
Dysmenorrhea	Uterus-I5; Internal Secretion-D1; Sympathetic-H1; Shen Men-I1.	
Amenorrhea	Uterus-I5; Internal Secretion-D1; Ovary-D2; Adrenal Gland-B8.	Adrenal Gland-B8.
Functional Hemorrhage from the Uterus	Uterus-I5; Brain-E4; Internal Secretion-D1; Liver-N9; Spleen-N10; Kidney-N4.	
Leukorrhagia	Uterus-I5; Ovary-D2; Internal Secretion-D1.	
Endometritis	Same as above, plus Adrenal Gland-B8.	External Genitalia-I10.
Prolapse of Uterus	Uterus-I5; Subcortex-E10.	External Genitalia-I10.
Chronic Pelvioperitonitis	Uterus-I1; Ovary-D2; Internal Secretion-D1; Pelvic Cavity-I2.	
Adnexitis	Ovary-D2; Internal Secretion-D1; Shen Men-I1.	Adrenal Gland-B8.
Postnatal Involution pain	Uterus-I5; Sympathetic-H1; Shen Men-I1.	Subcortex-E10.
Vulvar Pruritis	External Genitalia-I10 (pecking); Occiput-E5; Adrenal Gland-B8; Shen Men-I1; Lung-O2; Internal Secretion-D1.	

SUBJECT: OPHTHALMOLOGY

DISEASES	MAJOR POINTS	SECONDARY POINTS
Hordeolum; Chalazion	Eye-A10; Liver-N9; Spleen-N10.	
Acute Conjunctivitis	Eye-A10; Liver-N9.	
Anaphylatic Conjunctivitis	Eye-A10; Liver-N9; Occiput-E5; Internal Secretion-D1.	
Follicular Conjunctivitis	Eye-A10; Liver-N9.	
Electric Ophthalmitis	Kidney-N4; Liver-N9; Eye-A10.	Shen Men-I1.
Glaucoma (Devil's Eyes)	Kidney-N4; Liver-N9; Eye^1-D3; Eye^2-D4; Eye-A10.	
Papillitis	Same as above.	
Optic Atrophy	Kidney-N4; Liver-N9; Eye-A10.	
Night Blindness	Liver-N9; Eye^2-D4; Eye-A10.	
Myopia	Kidney-N4; Liver-N9; Eye^2-D4; Eye-A10.	
Diffused Light	Kidney-N4; Liver-N9; Eye-A10; Eye^2-D4; Occiput-E5.	
Diplopia	Kidney-N4; Liver-N9; Eye^2-D4; Eye-A10.	

SUBJECT: OTORHINOLARYNGOLOGY

DISEASES	MAJOR POINTS	SECONDARY POINTS
Tinnitis Aurium	Kidney-N4; Occiput-E5; Internal Ear-A12; External Ear-C1.	
Impaired Hearing	Kidney-N4; Occiput-E5; Internal Ear-A12; External Ear-C1.	
Furunculosis of the External Meatus	Kidney-N4; Internal Ear-A12; Internal Secretion-D1.	External Ear-C1.
Otitis Media	Kidney-N4; Internal Ear-A12; Internal Secretion-D1.	External Ear-C1.
Simple Rhinitis	Internal Nose-B6; Adrenal Gland-B8; Forehead-E9;	Lung-O2.
Atrophic Rhinitis	Same as above.	
Anaphylatic Rhinitis	Same as above, plus Internal Secretion-D1.	
Epistaxis	Internal Nose-B6; Adrenal Gland-B8; Forehead-E9.	
Ulcerous Vestibulum Nasi	Same as above, plus Lune-O2.	
Sinusitis	Internal Nose-B6; Adrenal Gland-B8; Forehead-E9.	
Chronic Pharyngitis	Pharynx & Larynx-B4; Shen Men-I1; Heart-O2; Internal Secretion-D1.	
Chronic Laryngitis	Same as above.	Lung-O2; Hou Ya-E3.
Hoarseness	Pharynx & Larynx-B4; Shen Men-I1; Heart-O1; Lung-O2.	Internal Secretion-D1.

Acute Tonsillitis	Tonsils[3]-A6; Pharynx & Larynx-B4.	Helix[1]-K1–Helix[6]-K6.
Uvular Oedema	Pharynx & Larynx-B4; Shen Men-I1; Adrenal Gland-B8.	

SUBJECT: STOMATOLOGY

DISEASES	MAJOR POINTS	SECONDARY POINTS
Decayed Teeth; Toothache	Maxilla-A7; Mandible-A5; Shen Men-I1; Toothache-E2.	Hou Ya-E3.
Periodontitis	Maxilla-A7; Mandible-A5; Mouth-M1; Adrenal Gland-B8.	Kidney-N4.
Retardation of the development of teeth	Maxilla-A7; Mandible-A5; Shen Men-I1; Toothache-E2.	Hou Ya-E3.
Agomphiasis	Kidney-N4; Mandible-A5; Maxilla-A7; Occiput-E5.	
Mouth Ulcer	Mouth-M1; Internal Secretion-D1; Shen Men-I1; Tougue-A3.	
Mycotic Stomatitis	Mouth-M1; Internal Secretion-D1; Adrenal Gland-B8; Spleen-N10; Occiput-E5.	
Glossitis	Tongue-A3; Mouth-M1; Internal Secretion-D1; Heart-01.	

SUBJECT: DERMATOLOGY

DISEASES	MAJOR POINTS	SECONDARY POINTS
Folliculitis; Herpes Zoster	Corresponding to area (pecking); Lung-O2; Occiput-E5; Internal Secretion-D1; Adrenal Gland-B8.	
Verruca Vulgaris	Lung-O2; Internal Secretion-D1; Occiput-E5; Adrenal Gland-B8; Corresponding to area (pecking).	
Pernio (1-2 degrees)	Corresponding to area; Shen Men-I1; Occiput-E5; Spleen-N10; Adrenal Gland-B8.	
Dermatitis Solaris	Shen Men-I1; Lung-O2; Internal Secretion-D1; Adrenal Gland-B8.	
Exzema; Verrucaplana	Lung-O2; Internal Secretion-D1; Occiput-E5; Large Intestine-M8.	
Infantile Eczema	Corresponding to area; Lung-O2; Occiput-E5; Internal Secretion-D1.	
Anaphylactic Dermatitis	Lung-O2; Internal Secretion-D1; Occiput-E5; Adrenal Gland-B8; Corresponding to area (pecking).	
Urticaria	Lung-O2; Shen Men-I1; Occiput-E5; Internal Secretion-D1; Adrenal Gland-B8.	
Cutaneous Pruritus	Shen Men-I1; Lung-O2; Occiput-E5; Internal Secretion-D1; Adrenal Gland-B8.	
Neurodermatitis	Corresponding to area (pecking); Occiput-E5; Internal Secretion-D1; Adrenal Gland-B8.	

Condition	Points
Chorionitis	Lung-O2; Occiput-E5; Internal Secretion-D1; Adrenal Gland-B8; Liver-N9; Spleen-N10; Brain-E4.
Dermatitis Seborrhoica	Lung-O2; Internal Secretion-D1; Spleen-N10; Occiput-E5; Adrenal Gland-B8.
Vitiligo	Lung-O2; Internal Secretion-D1; Occiput-E5; Adrenal Gland-B8; corresponding to area (pecking).
Alopecia	Kidney-N4; Lung-O2; Internal Secretion-D1; Occiput-E5.
Alopecia Areata	Corresponding to area (pecking); Kidney-N4; Lung-O2; Internal Secretion-D1.
Acne	Lung-O2; Internal Secretion-D1; Testicle-E8; Cheeks-A11 (pecking).
Rosacea	External Nose-B5 (pecking); Lung-O2; Internal Secretion-D1; Adrenal Gland-B8.
Miliaria	Lung-O2; Internal Secretion-D1; Adrenal Gland-B8; Occiput-E5; Shen Men-I1.

SUBJECT: ADDITIONAL

DISEASES	MAJOR POINTS	SECONDARY POINTS
Heat Stroke	Occiput-E5; Heart-O1; Subcortex-E10; Adrenal Gland-B8.	
Seasickness; Trainsickness	Occiput-E5; Stomach-M4.	Internal Ear-A12; Shen Men-I1.
Edema with indistinct origin	Kidney-N4; Bladder-N1; Heart-O1; Liver-N9; Sympathetic-H1; Internal Secretion-D1.	
Low Grade Fever without Distinct Origin	Apex of Auricle-K12; Apex of Tragus-B1; Adrenal Gland-B8 (blood-letting); Internal Secretion-D1; Liver-N9; Spleen-N10; Shen Men-I1.	
Multiple Lymphnodoncus	Ku Kuan-I3; Occiput-E5; Internal Secretion-D1.	

DIAGRAM 10
French foetal representation

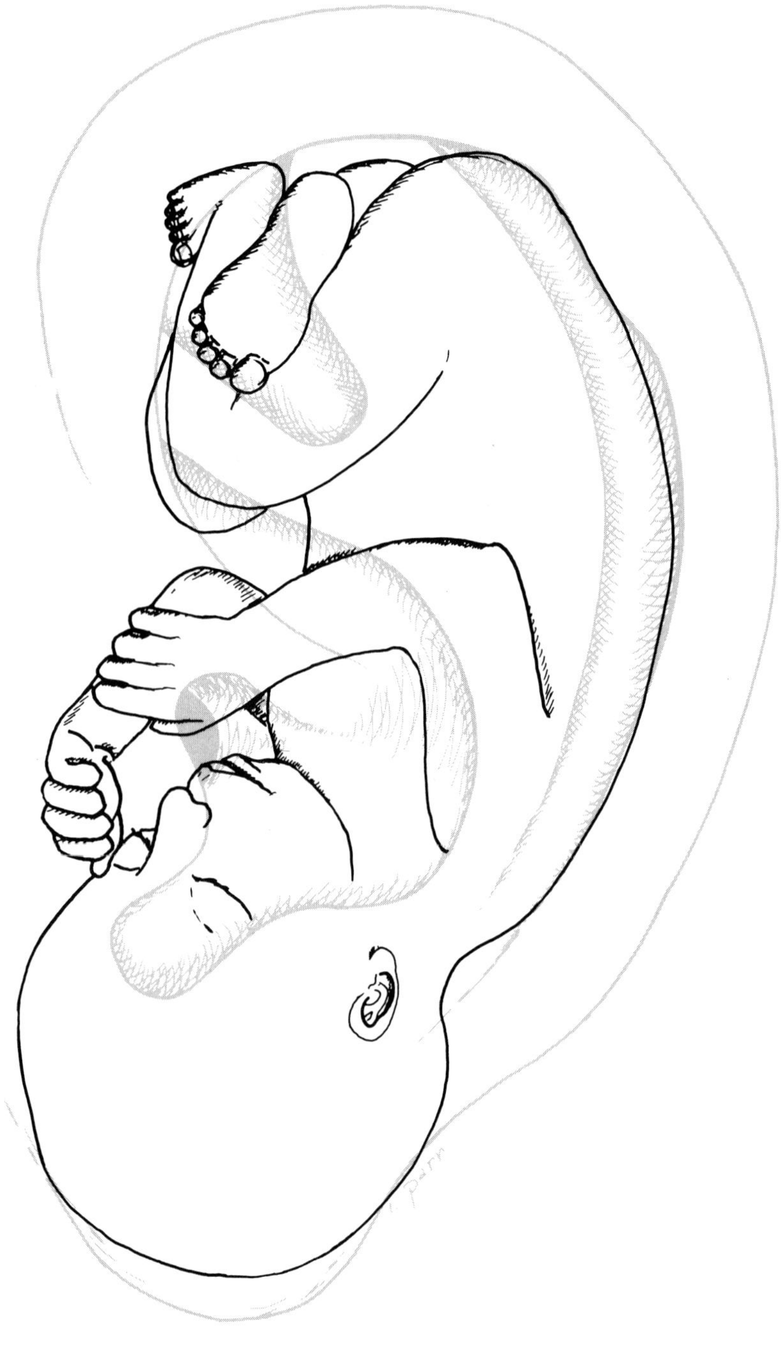

CHAPTER 10

DR. NOGIER'S POINTS

The reader may find it curious to note that many of Dr. Nogier's points are situated differently than the Chinese points. My aim is not to praise either the Chinese or Dr. Nogier, though both are worthy of much praise, but to mark these differences, that you may better use the ear for treatment. There are no doubt many reasons for these differences from one author and scientist to another. In this case one of the obvious reasons lies in the different location and position that each gives the limbs of the foetus to which, as you know by now, the ear corresponds. (see Diagram 10.)

It is obvious that one should be tempted to prefer the Chinese ear points, knowing that the Chinese have at their command thousands of researchers in every possible area. Nevertheless, most acupuncturists who have used the ear for their treatments, would agree that in many cases, Nogier's points give better results. Besides, and I will again repeat myself, the Chinese are the first to acknowledge Dr. Nogier as the "Father of Ear Acupuncture".

Although I shall describe some of the important characteristics of Nogier's method, at no time am I pretending to expose it in its entirety. For those of you who are familiar with his book entitled "Treatise of Auriculotherapy", you will understand that in a volume of this considerable size he exposed but a brief part of his extensive knowledge on this subject.

A) The Antihelix, the Key to Dr. Nogier's Ear Chart:

The antihelix of the auricle corresponds to the spinal column. The posterior auricular sulcus corresponds to the space between the atlas and the occipital shell. From there upwards on the antihelix, to the end of the lower crurae of the antihelix, in a semicircle, we have the different levels of the vertebral column, starting from the cervical to sacral and coccygeal. (Diagram 11). The key points to retain in this area are those corresponding to the first and last vertebrae of each vertebral level. These are C1 (1st cervical, or Atlas), C7 (7th cervical), D1 (1st dorsal), D12 (12th dorsal), L1 (1st lumbar), L5 (5th lumbar); S1 (1st sacral).

This will be helpful in all treatments, as we shall soon see. With Point Zero as a point of reference, a line can be drawn from this point through the vertebrae and extended to the helix. This helps us to locate precisely the different parts of the limbs (see diagram 12). Also the limbs are thus connected to the spinal column. This is not a chance relationship but has proven experimentally to be valid.

To further illustrate these alignments I will give a few examples. Let us say that a patient complains of pain in the region of the 1st lumbar vertebra. Normally, needling the L1 point will relieve the pain. In this case it doesn't work. A line is drawn from Point Zero through the 1st Lumbar point and extended to the helix. It will generally be found that along this line, and at regular intervals (called "Steps"), other painful spots are present. Needling these points will often relieve the pain and effect a cure. (see Diagram 13). The alignment of points on such radii is exact to about a 1mm error. Any such radius may be extended through to the helix from Point Zero, once one painful spot has been found anywhere.

There are other such alignments which are effective. Let us take radius OA as reference. We can then draw a line AB at 30 degrees to OA above it and a line AD at 30 degrees below it. These lines will generally hold other painful spots once radius OA has been determined. (see Diagram 13).

B) The Lobule:

The lobule is the part of the ear which commands con-

ditioned reflexes. For instance, someone who has been im-
mobilized for a long time, say, in a cast or a wheelchair may not
be able to move about even once the damage seems repaired. Simply needling points corresponding to parts of the body that are
deficient does not produce positive results. In this case one often
finds that it is a "visual image" that "I cannot walk" or I cannot
possibly move my arm now" that is hindering recovery. This is a
conditioned reflex.

Dr. Nogier divides the lobule into four zones. a Visual
Zone, an Auditory Zone, an Olfactory Zone, and an Intellectual
Zone (see Diagram 14a). One point controls all these zones; this
point is called the Sensorial point. These zones deal with conditioned reflexes. Thus according to whether it is a visual image (I
cannot see myself walking), an auditory image (I hear my joints
cracking), an olfactory image, (I have sinusitis, therefore I cannot
possibly smell anything), or a rationalization, that is causing this
conditioned reflex, the corresponding zones of the lobule are controlled for pain referral both anteriorly and posteriorly and the
proper treatment is administered.

C) The Root of the Helix:

This area commands the emotions. It is used for patients
who do not have a particular image hindering their progress, but
when it is anxiety that is blocking them. Such patients are easily
identifiable in that they are always anxious and no matter how
much they improve they are still afraid.

The zone to be dealt with here is a zone extending from
Point Zero to the medial aspect of the antihelix, at about the 3rd
Cervical area. This line corresponds to the sympathetic plexi from
the navel (point Zero) to the carotidian plexus (Marvellous Point).
The Marvellous point is so named because of its effectiveness in
treating Hypertension. (see Diagram 15).

D) The Tragus:

Both tragi correspond to different bodily tissues. What the
left tragus represents to a right-handed person is the opposite to a
southpaw. The same is true of the right tragus.

For a right-handed person, the left tragus reacts on the
osteoarticular and muscular systems. The right tragus reacts on

the vegetative functions. The opposite is true for a left-handed person. (see Diagrams 16a & 16b).

POINT ZERO AND GLANDULAR CONTROL POINTS*

Point Zero: This point is the geometric and physiological center of the outer ear, from which the various segments can be located with precision. It is to be found at the root of the antihelix, in a notch which can easily be felt with the fingers. It is painful in almost all ailments. This point is to be used when there is an absence of pain referral on the auricle. Needling of this point in such cases will bring about a response and immediate pain referral on the auricle or peripheral disorders. Similarly, when there are too many painful spots on the ear, this point will eliminate all but the essential reactive points.

Glandular Control Points:

A) **Hypothalamus point:** It is situated in the concha, at the foot of the antitragus, where a depressed ridge is felt by pressing with the finger. It acts on the entire homologous side of the body . . . arm, leg, face, skin surface, without affecting the spinal column. Thus diseases as varied as arthritis, spasms, paralysis, and skin diseases can be treated by this point.

B) **Genital Point:** It is situated at the spot where the ridge of the antihelix meets the intertragic incisure and about 1mm. down from it, on the lobule. It is effective in all gonadic disorders, more so in women than in men, and also in treating the joints and skin.

C) **Surrenalian Point:** It is located on the opposite side of the intertragic incisure from the Genital point, at the base of the tragus. It is effective in stimulating energy and regulating blood pressure. It also serves in treating the spinal column and limbs when other points are insufficient.

---

*See diagram 14b, & 17.

D) **Thyroidian & Parathyroidian Points:** They are situated inside the notch formed by the intertragic incisure, at about 1mm.'s distance from each other. The Thyroidian point is closer to the edge of the incisure, whereas the Parathyroidian point is situated a little deeper. They are most effective in joint pain and in calcic disorders.

THE AURICULO-CARDIAC REFLEX

This reflex (known as the ACR reflex) is an extremely valuable means of diagnosis and offers perhaps the key to a true understanding of acupuncture in general, not only ear acupuncture.

I had been using a similar method with normal body acupuncture long before I heard of Dr. Nogier. I compare my method to a lie detector test. Instead of using a galvanometer, as is normally done by the police, I use the pulse. It had always been my firm belief that every patient is aware, at least subconsciously, what his troubles really are. Whatever disease he is suffering from is due to the inability to bring to the surface or consciousness this deep subconscious knowledge. Of course I am merely emitting a hypothesis here, which though it has proven correct for myself in treating thousands of patients, may seem absurd to someone else. In any case, Avicenna, to whom we owe a great deal in the field of medicine, used the pulse in the same way.

Dr. Nogier's Auriculo-Cardiac Reflex will not be dealt with in great detail here. My aim is only to arouse your curiosity so that some of you may seek to familiarize yourselves with his work. In my opinion the importance of his work will not be realized or bear fruit for another century or so, as it is the launching pad of a new insight into mankind.

To measure the ACR, the physician must place himself behind the patient. Both the physician and the patient should be in a comfortable and relaxed position. With one hand the patient's pulse is felt; not the deep pulse, but the more superficial beats. The patient's arm must not be twisted painfully. At the same time, the auricle is palpated with a probe which should be as neutral as possible, that is, neither hot, nor cold, nor humid. For this purpose, a cork-tipped probe is best.

Once a point is stimulated slightly with the probe, the physician must wait a few beats, disregarding a change in the first few beats. Only after 4-10 beats have gone by, is it noted if there is an increase or decrease of the pulse rhythm. The amount of time it takes for the pulse to return to normal, after the initial change is called the "period of Latency". This period of latency serves to determine whether the patient has the constitution required of him to recover quickly, or hasn't, and the degree of traumatism involved.

After the point has been tested with the neutral probe, a lukewarm probe, and then a cold probe are used. Whichever of these probes serves to deteriorate or to correct the pulse rhythm most rapidly is used for reference in the treatment. For example, if the rhythm was regularized by a warm probe, but deteriorated by a cold one, then a gold needle or a positive current can regulate the problem. If the ACR was slowed down by a warm probe and improved by a cold one, then we should use a silver needle or a negative current. If both warm and cold have the same effect, then a stainless steel needle will be used.

As can be clearly seen, when one envisages all the points on the auricle examined in this way, the process may be a lengthy one, taking as much as one or two hours for one patient. It can, however, come in very handy in certain difficult cases which seem impossible to diagnose correctly no matter which tests are administered.

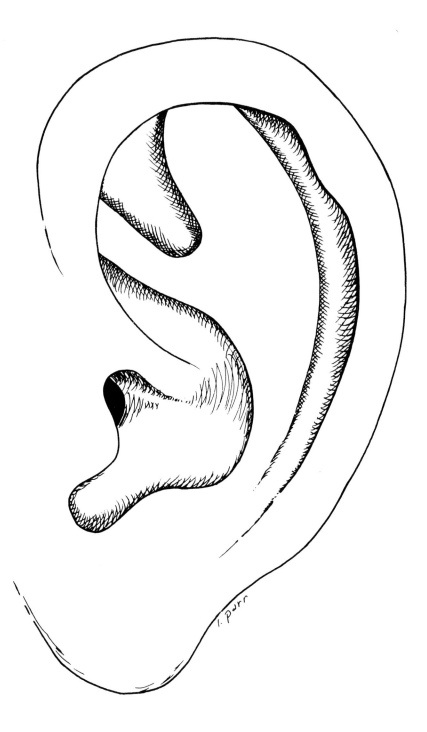

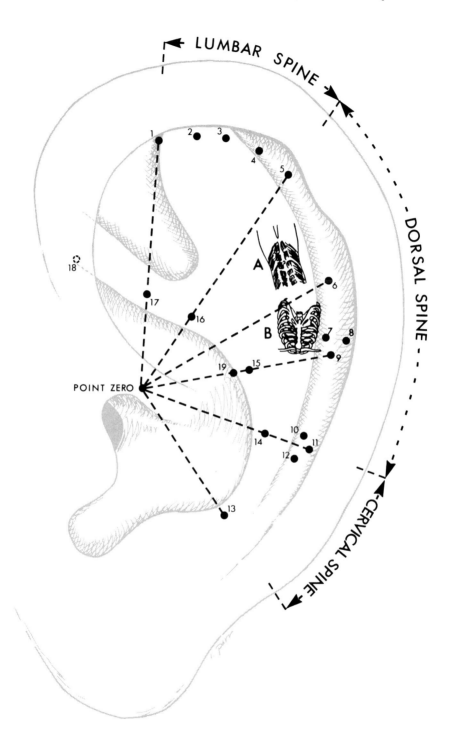

DIAGRAM 11

Auricular projections of spinal cord, upper limb, and scapular girdle, and how they are linked through point Zero.

   1. thumb
   2. index finger
   3. middle finger
   4. ring finger
   5. little finger
   6. wrist
   7. radius
   8. ulnar
   9. elbow
  10. clavicle
  11. shoulder
  12. scapula
  13. atlas
  14. 7th cervical vertebra
  15. 5th dorsal vertebra
  16. 1st lumbar vertebra
  17. 5th lumbar vertebra
  18. coccyx
  19. breast
   B. sternum & rib cage

   A. abdominal muscles

DIAGRAM 12

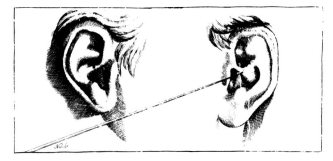

Extract from old French manuscript indicating use of ears for treating various illnesses ranging from toothache to sciatica. One single treatment was said to suffice to alleviate pain for several years, to life.

DIAGRAM 13
Steps and Radii

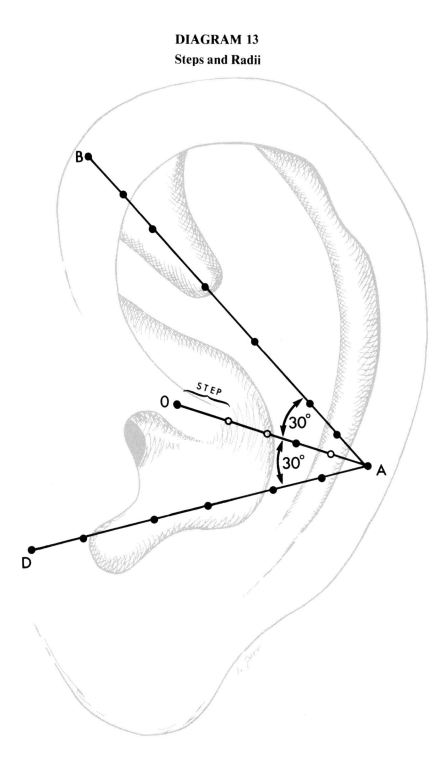

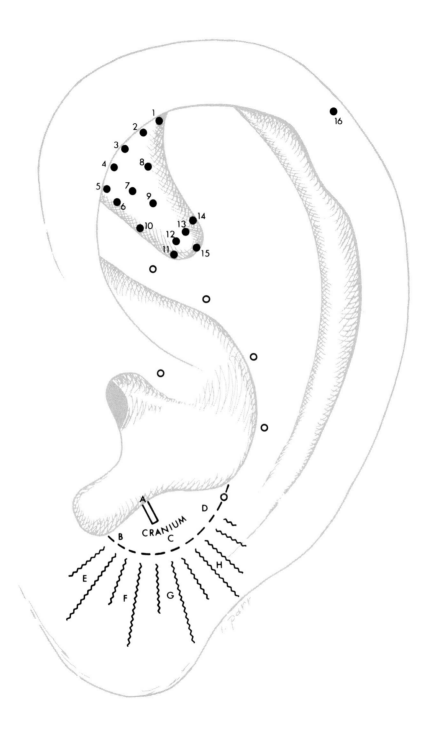

DIAGRAM 14a
Zones of the lobule and antitragus (antitragus = cranium).
Lower limb projections in the triangular fossa.

1. halux toe
2. 2nd toe
3. 3rd toe
4. 4th toe
5. 5th toe
6. heel
7. internal malleolus
8. external malleolus
9. knee
10. sciatica point
11. sacro-iliac
12. buttocks
13. Scarpa's triangle
14. pubic symphysis
15. hip (coxo-femoral joint)
16. Coxalgia point

A. Tic line
B. frontal bone
C. temples
D. occiput
E. Intellectual zone
F. Olfactory zone
G. Auditive zone
H. Visual zone

∿∿∿∿ = energetic projections from the antitragus (cranium) into the lobule.

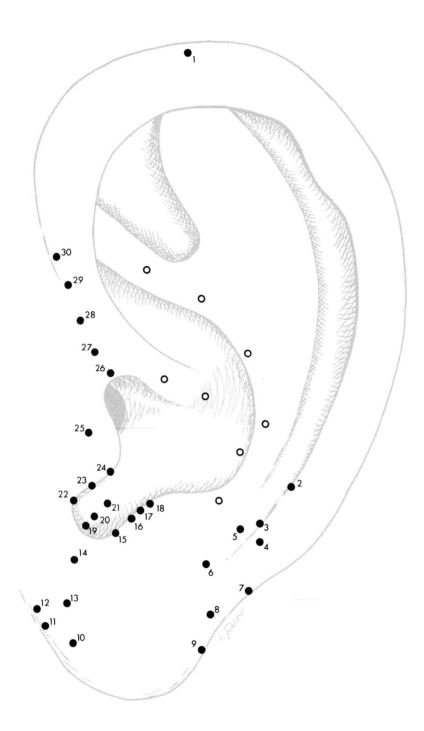

DIAGRAM 14b
**Lobule points. Antitragus and tragus glandular control points.
External genito-urinary organs on ascending branch of the helix.**

1. allergy point
2. diminishing libido point.
3. temporo-maxillary joint
4. mandible
5. maxillary
6. sensorial point⁻
7. metabolic regulation point
8. Joy point
9. sneezing point
10. tooth analgesia²
11. headache point
12. Agressivity point
13. Omega point
14. tooth analgesia¹
15. genital point
16. sleeping point
17. antihypophysis
18. Hypothalamus
19. parathyroid
20. thyroid
21. thymus
22. suprarenal gland
23. mammary gland
24. thermoregulation point
25. vitality point (cancer)
26. Exciting libido point (glans penis—glans clitoridis)
27. urethra
28. labia minora—prepuce
29. labia majorascrotum
30. anus

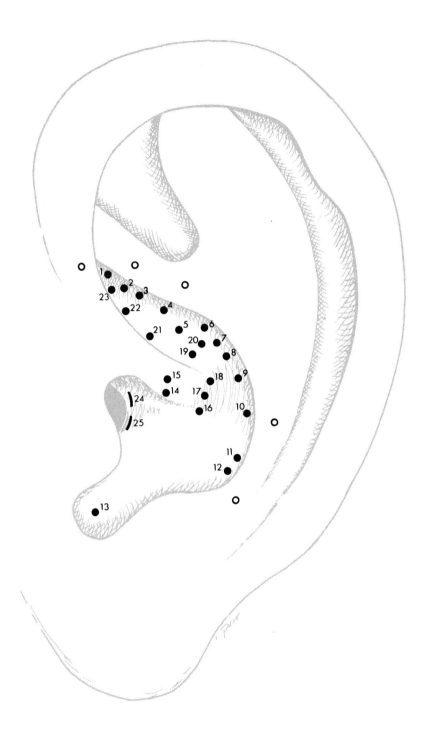

DIAGRAM 15
Concha projections of internal organs and control points.

1., 2., 3. left colon
4. right colon
5. gall bladder
6. ileum
7. jejunum
8. duodenum
9. stomach
10. inferior cervical ganglia
11. marvellous point (5th thoracic vertebra).
12. heart (3rd-4th thoracic vertebrae)
13. thyroid
14. hypogastric plexus[2]
15. point Zero (hypogastric plexus)
16. 6th thoracic vertebra.
17. Solar plexus (7th thoracic vertebra)
18. splanchnic nerve
19. liver
20. pancreas
21. bladder
22. ureter
23. kidney
24. respiratory functions
25. cardiac functions

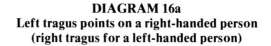

DIAGRAM 16a
Left tragus points on a right-handed person
(right tragus for a left-handed person)

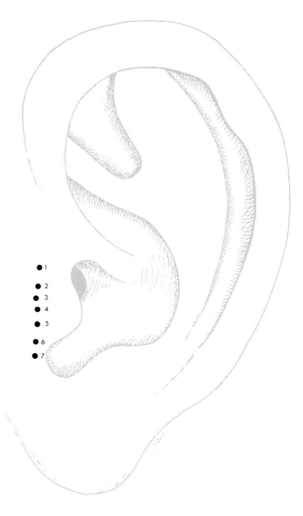

1. coccyx
2. sacrum
3. lumbar vertebrae
4. thoracic vertebrae

5. thoracic vertebrae
6. cervical vertebrae
7. cranium & head

DIAGRAM 16b
Right tragus points on a right-handed person
(left tragus for a left-handed person)

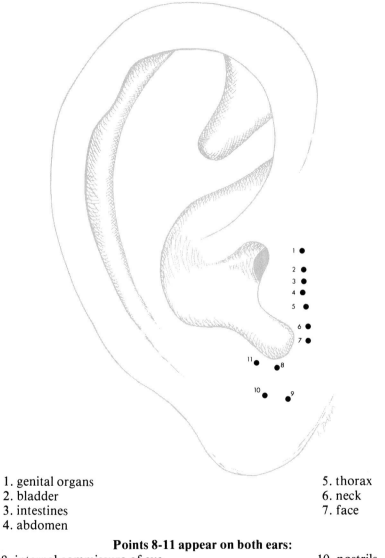

1. genital organs   5. thorax
2. bladder   6. neck
3. intestines   7. face
4. abdomen

Points 8-11 appear on both ears:

8. internal commissura of eye   10. nostrils
9. external commissura of eye   11. root of nose

DIAGRAM 17
Points around the external acoustic meatus
and on the inside of the tragus. Various regulatory centers

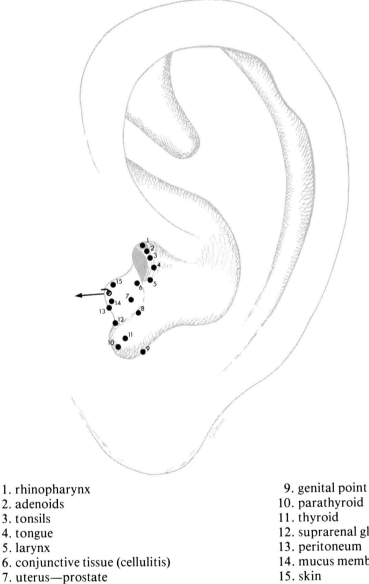

1. rhinopharynx
2. adenoids
3. tonsils
4. tongue
5. larynx
6. conjunctive tissue (cellulitis)
7. uterus—prostate
8. thermoregulation point
9. genital point
10. parathyroid
11. thyroid
12. suprarenal gland
13. peritoneum
14. mucus membranes
15. skin

DIAGRAM 18
Points appearing on the back of the Auricle

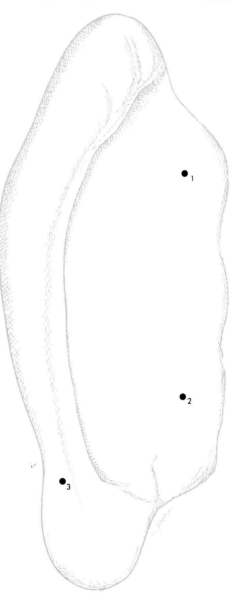

1. Ear disorders (back of knee point)
2. Respiratory function point
3. Sciatica point (back of temporo-maxillary joint point)

WEXU EAR POINTS

The following is a list of points which I have discovered through my daily practice to give good results. The first time I attended a Nogier seminar on Auriculotherapy I was amazed that the ear could be used to treat so many diseases. Naturally my first reaction was one of scepticism. Nevertheless, I proceeded to experiment on myself whenever I wasn't feeling well and little by little I became convinced that indeed Nogier had discovered something of great value to humanity. My research also led me to the discovery of several zones on the ear that Nogier does not mention.

1) **Self-identity zone (Pan's Point):** I have named this point after the Greek God Pan because in musically inclined people, this zone is either pointed, giving the ear a pointed appearance, or else the cartilage is hardened in this area. In my opinion it is a point that serves to strengthen the character of the individual, in order that he might further express his personal talents.

2) **Hypothalamus Control Zone:** Needling this area subcutaneously along its length, approximately 1/2 inch, and directing the needle from the front to the back of the auricle, gives good results in physical disorders of a degenerative nature. The needle must either be twirled manually for a few seconds, up to one minute, and then again after five more minutes, or else an electrical current can be applied for 10 minutes up to one half hour. One may also combine the manual twirling with the electrical stimulation.

3) **Wei Qi command zone:** As you know, the helix of the auricle corresponds to the back of the fetus and therefore to the Yang (positive) energy. This implies that the helix commands the Wei Qi, or defensive energy of the body. In my comparison of the auricle to a micro-castle (see Chapter 3) the helix corresponds to the outer fortification of the castle, which is synonymous to the Chinese viewpoint.

People who have a deteriorated helix are chronically sick people. Whichever part of the helix is deteriorated indicates that the corresponding peripheral area of the body is in poor condition. As a matter of fact this part of the body was used since ancient times in China to examine the state of the body's defences.

I have found the auricular tubercle (Darwin's tubercle) to be the zone of the ear that serves to strengthen the body's defenses, and opens the helix to receive a flux of energy.

4) **Alertness Points:** These points are situated one below the other on the helix, slightly below the Wei Qi point. They serve to strengthen the action of the Hypothalamus control point and should be used in conjunction with it.

5) **Triceps point (aggressivity):** This point is close to the classical Lumbo-sacral region. I have correlated this point to the Triceps muscles in that the Triceps are the muscles that give us strength in pushing objects. No doubt this reflex begins at the lumbo-sacral region, but it finds its energetic outlet in the Triceps. In people having naturally developed Triceps it will be found that this area is well developed.

6) **Arthritis and calcic disorder control zone:** The arthritis zone is situated along both sides of the crus of the helix. The Calcic zone forms the crest of this former zone.

These areas, when stimulated mildly, first by massage (with the cap of a fountain pen for instance) and then by electricity, are effective in treating most forms of arthritis.

7) **Cosmic Receptivity Zone and Control Point:** I have found, and no doubt I am not the only one, that the lobule of the ear is the area which acts as a receptor for cosmic messages, or ideas as they are called. This explains the stimulating effect of touch or caresses in this area and is also the reason sailors, Sufi priests and even women wear earrings. Stimulation of the lobule and its control point is particularly effective with intellectuals and weak-minded people, and in treating psychosomatic disorders, depressions and suicidal tendencies. A mild electrical current may be used in the latter case.

8) **Relaxing zone:** This zone is effective in diminishing stress.

9) **Mineral metabolism point:** This point is very close to the classical Shen Men point. It is useful for treating intellectuals who are overworking themselves.

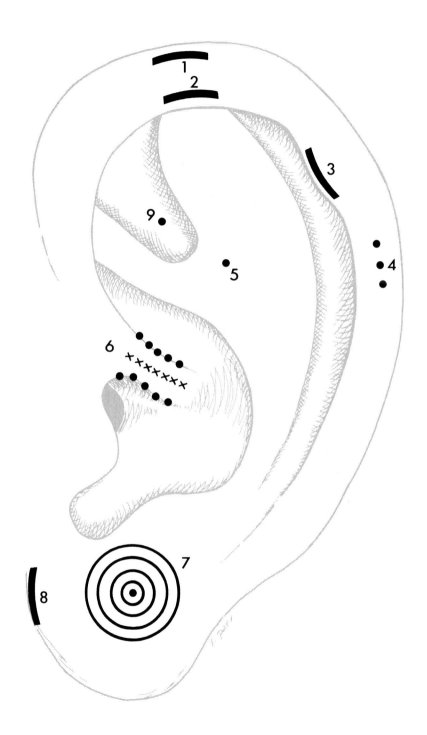

DIAGRAM 19
Wexu points.

1. Self-identity Zone (Pan point)
2. Hypothalamus Control Zone
3. Wei Qi Command Zone
4. Alertness Zone & Points
5. Triceps Point (agressivity)
6. Arthritis and Calcic disorder zones
7. Cosmic receptivity (intuition, intellectual) zone and control point
8. Relaxing zone
9. Mineral metabolism point

SECTION IV:

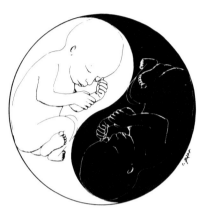

Special Applications

CHAPTER 11

DRUG ADDICTION, ALCOHOLISM AND NICOTINE ADDICTION

a) **Drug Addiction:**

Nothing is more effective in treating tension in whatever form it may present itself than acupuncture. The withdrawal symptoms of a person addicted to a hard drug include violent fits of tension, accompanied by nausea, headache, chills, vomiting, sensitivity to light, to name a few.

By reducing the tension proportionately to each individual by means of acupuncture, the body can disintoxicate itself more rapidly and adjust to the environment. Recent research in this field,* carried out in Hong Kong at the Kwong Wah hospital through the initiative of S.Y.C. Cheung of the Neurological Division, indicate that such treatment is possible. An average of two months after initial treatment is necessary to completely disintoxicate the patient and rid him of any traces of the drug that he was taking. Similar results are being obtained now in many countries and in the U.S.A. and Canada as well.

The treatment is a simple one, but because of individual differences in behavior patterns, it is often necessary to intern the

---

*Reported in May 1973 Drugs & Society Vol. 2 #8.

patient for at least the first week or two of treatment. Many patients require 2-3 treatments per day in the beginning and an acupuncturist must be present 24 hours a day, ready to administer treatment whenever the withdrawal symptoms present themselves. This is of vital importance in the beginning because the acupuncture needles and stimulation are evaluated by the patient in terms of a substitute for the drug. Some patients seem completely cured after only two or three treatments and lab tests show them to be drug free, but this is far from being the general rule.

Generally, once there is the slightest improvement of the patient's condition, the treatments can be spread out to every two days and then to every three days and so on. The patient himself will tell you of the value of the treatment compared to a certain dose of drugs. The psychological element is relatively small, as most patients treated in this way were highly sceptical as to this type of treatment.

The Technique

The patient lies on his back on a bed or table. The points to be needled are situated on the hands, forearms and ears. Now nose points are being used to replace the points on the arms. The points are as follows:

> —Ho-ku (LI 4) to a depth of 1cm.
> —Hou-hsi (SI 3) to a depth of 0.5cm.
> —Wai-kuan (TB 5) to a depth of 1cm.
> —Nei-kuan (EH 6) to a depth of 2.5cm.
> —Shen-men (He 7) to a depth of 0.5cm.

Ear points:
—Nao Kan (Brain axis point—E1)
—Nao Tien (Brain point—E4).

The two ear points, which are very close together, are pierced obliquely, subcutaneously for 1/2 cm., slanting towards the base of the concha.

The needles are then attached by wires to an electrical stimulator which can produce a current of up to 35 V., and has a frequency range of up to 200 impulses per second. Voltage and frequency must be controlled at all times and either increased or decreased, according to the reactions of the patient. They must be adjusted individually to each patient. Stimulation is usually maintained from 20 minutes to three quarters of an hour, though quite often the patient will state that he feels better after only 10-15 minutes of stimulation. He will complain of such symptoms as dryness of eyes, nose and mouth, but will add that he feels warmer and can breathe well and would like a cup of coffee. This is a sign that the treatment is producing good results and therefore the electrical stimulation must be stopped.

Another reaction is that the patient feels a sudden urge to urinate. Again this is interpreted as a good reaction and stimulation must be stopped and the patient allowed to relax and relieve himself.

Upon observing the patient it will be found that he is more sociable and less neurotic in that the desire to alienate himself has gone.

Another method which some acupuncturists are using, probably through personal initiative, is pecking the forearm with the needle for a few minutes before actually inserting it in the Lung 7 point or Heart 3 or 7. This method seems to yield very good results as well.

Today the number of needles have been greatly reduced and only 4 needles are necessary, one in each ear and one in each arm. The ear point is the Lung point (02). The left Lung point is deemed more effective and can be used alone. The needle must be inserted under the skin, towards the external auditory canal for a length of 1/2 inch. Another needle is inserted at Ho-ku (LI 4) and an electrical stimulation maintained for about 1/2 hour at a frequency of 140-160 impulses per second. It seems that the ear points are the most effective. Almost any body point can be used, but if the ear is not used the results are not as good.

Advantages of this type of treatment

Treating drug addicts by a natural method such as acupuncture undoubtably must be preferred over methadone maintenance, which consists of merely addicting the patient to another drug. Acupuncture is cheap, effective and produces no side effects. Obviously this does not obviate the necessity of maintaining social work, and psychiatry. It would be most profitable both for the patient and for the national budget in health care to consider instituting this type of treatment in the near future.

b) **Alcoholism and nicotine addiction**

Alcoholism:

The procedure is similar to the one employed in drug addiction. The points on the arm may remain the same: He 3,7, EH 6, TB 5, LI 4, One point on the lower extremities may be added: Li 3. The ear points are indicated in the appendix in the chapter dealing with the treatment of diseases of the mental and nervous system. Points along the nose and mouth can be used at times to replace other distal points on the arms or legs. We have obtained good results in our clinic in Montreal without having to intern the patient, though no doubt severe cases need internment for the first few weeks of treatment.

Nicotine addiction:

Again only the ear points change. As to the distal points, Zu San-li (St 36), and Lung 5 can be used alternately with other points. The ear points are indicated in the appendix under the same heading as the above.

N.B. In all three cases mentioned above it will be noticed that whatever other disease the patient was suffering from, such as asthma, ulcers, backache, migraine, will also disappear.

OBESITY

Contrary to what is advocated by many acupuncturists, there is no miracle cure for obesity. Acupuncture certainly helps people to lose weight, but quite gradually, by renormalizing the flow of energy of the body. It seems that no matter what type of ailment is treated, an overweight patient will also lose weight as his general condition improves.

Obesity due to nervous causes responds quite well to acupuncture therapy, as well as abdominal distention due to gas or constipation. If there is a glandular cause to the disorder, it will be more difficult to effect a cure, since many nervous centers are affected simultaneously and the condition is usually more deep rooted.

One type of treatment has gained quick popularity in North America in recent years. This is the staple treatment for obesity. The machine used is sold at a very expensive price and is nothing more than a surgical suture machine. This method has nothing to do with acupuncture. A staple is implanted in the ear in over-weight patients and maintained in place for as long as one week or ten days. Whenever the patient thinks about eating he is to rub the staple and this will calm his appetite. This sounds very nice. There is one inconvenience; the risk of losing your ear if it gets infected.

It is quite possible that this method may have brought about some good results, but I am curious to know if this is not due to the traumatism that this staple causes. The patient who has such a staple in his ear cannot sleep on that side of his head and must pay constant attention that no one will accidentally rub or touch his ear. This becomes quite irritating in the long run and especially if there is an infection to any degree, the patient will lose weight. As you know, the cartilage of the ear has no defences, and a thick foreign body will tend to cause infection. The strongest resistance to infection is at the level of the skin.

I must point out that these staples are not the same as the minute Chinese permanent tack-like needles. Even with the Chinese needles there is a risk of infection, though much smaller than with the staples. Another aspect of the staple method which I find rather strange, is that two points can be pierced together which are contradictory to each other. Unless the person who is applying them knows alot about ear needling therapy, this can be a great disadvantage in that it may overstimulate the patient.

It is quite normal that in a country where overweight is the rule, any method which purports to cure it will gain in popularity. The truth is, however, that nothing short of simultaneously calming the nerves and maintaining a diet will cure this national plague. I can recommend normal acupuncture, ear acupuncture or even the Chinese press needles and the ion-spheres for this purpose. They are not dangerous. There is some risk with the small

Chinese permanent press needles, and it is the acupuncturist's duty to warn the patient of any possible sign that may indicate infection.

A) Nervous origin:

—Brain point—E4
—Occiput—E5
—Dermis (subcortex)—E10
—Diaphragm—L1
—Stomach—M4
—Shen Men—I1
—Lungs—02

The above points need not be needled at the same time. Shen Men, however, should be used in each treatment.

B) Liver malfunction:

—Liver—N9
—Gall Bladder—N6
—Pancreas—N6
—Stomach—M4
—Occiput—E5
—Vertex—E12
—Nogier's Metabolism Control point
—Point Zero (Nogier point)

C) Glandular disorders:

—Hormone point—D1
—Hypothalamus point—(Nogier point)
—Brain—E4
—Testicle or Ovary—E8
—Sympathetic—H1
—Thyroid—F9
—Omega point (Nogier point)

CHAPTER 12

OTITIS—OTALGIA—DEAFNESS

This chapter does not deal with what is known strictly as "ear acupuncture", but explains more exclusively "acupuncture of the ears". Not very much information is available thus far in English of the methods used in acupuncture to treat various ear problems such as ear pain, inflammation or numerous forms of deafness. Yet acupuncture yields outstanding results in this area as ascertained by Chinese scientists and as we have also proven in our clinic in Montreal, Canada.

We have a free clinic for children who are born deaf, where under the approval of the Institute for the Deaf and Dumb (L'Institut des Sourds et Muets) of Montreal we treat these children ranging from the ages of 7 to 17, once a week, every Saturday. Although the Chinese say that such a large interval is insufficient to produce results, we have had outstanding success even after very few treatments. The results are measured by the children's physicians and those of the Institution. They have not been published yet as we are doing them only on an experimental basis and need more time to reach any definite conclusions. However we have had results indicating as much as 40% improvement after 5 to 10 treatments in a few cases. The average improvement after 10 treatments at weekly intervals is of the order of 15%. Very few have had no results at all and I suspect that in the near future should we be able to administer several treatments per week as they do in China, our results will serve to verify the Chinese ones. These methods will be described towards the end of this chapter. First of all I propose to expose the theories concerning the ears and their treatment as explained in some of the Chinese classics, in some cases a western physiological explanation, and to discuss the New Points that modern Chinese acupuncturists are using effectively today.

A) **The Ears in General:*** In the Yi Sio Jiu Men (Doorway to Medical Studies) a Chinese book published in 1575 by Li Yen, it is stated that the main and controlling point in treating the ears is *Ho-ku,* the source point of the Large Intestine meridian (LI 4). This point was deemed one of the strongest points of the body and thus applicable to the ears as well. In other words no matter which local points were used, the results would not be as good, nor as permanent if LI 4 was not used as well.

Another Chinese classic, known as the *Chen Chiu Ta Cheng* (Compendium of Acupuncture and Moxa) published towards 1600, has *Fung-ch'ih* Gall Bladder 20 as one of the main points for treating the ears, especially if an irridiation within the ear is felt on pressure. The Japanese also considered this point, because of its action on the sympathetic and vagus nerves, as a primary point. Its name, however, translated as "wind pond" would lead us to believe that this point is more useful in ear troubles arising through external causes, such as humidity or wind.

The Japanese use primarily *T'ien-chu,* Bladder 10, because of its favorable action on the vagus nerve and glossopharyngeal nerve which helps to activate the mucus membrane, the tongue, pharynx, eustachian tube, tympanum, all interconnected with hearing. Its name, translated as Sky Pillar, denotes its role in balancing mental and physical energy.

The Japanese further state that if pressure on the ear is felt within the inner ear and as far as the pharynx, *Yi-fung,* "Shielding from the Wind", TB 17 must be used, in conjunction

---

*See diagram 20 for acupuncture points mentioned in this chapter until the heading for *Deafness.*

with GB 20. No doubt, if the pressure is felt in the pharynx, the ear trouble is due to a cold or to the wind as the name implies. This point is located behind the base of the auricle which serves in fact as a screen from the wind.

If there is inflammation of the middle ear, the Japanese advocate the use of *Ting-hui* (listening conference), which is Gall Bladder 12, *Wan-gu*, (last bone) Gall Bladder 12, and *Nao-hu* (brain window) Governing Vessel 17. For an inflammation of the external ear, they recommend to needle *Ehr-men* (ear gate) or Triple Burner #21.

The 16th century Chinese classic, the *Yi Sio Jiu Men* recommends to apply the needle in dispersion at *Ting-hui* Gall Bladder 2, and *Yi-fung* Triple Burner 17 in such ear troubles as involving deafness, glandular disfunctions or pain, pruritus or abcesses.

B) Ear Cerumen:

This is known in Chinese as Ting Ting-ning. It may be an allusion to the noises that can arise from having wax in the ears. For its treatment, references in Japanese books, in the *Chen Chiu Tan Cheng,* and in *Yi Sio Jiu Men* all indicate the point *T'ing-kung-* (listening palace), Small Intestine #19. A later book, published in 1919 in Shanghai by a group of medical doctors, the *Chen Chiu Yi Che* (Easy Understanding of Acupuncture and Moxibustion) recommend using *Ting-hui* (GB 2), *Yi-fung* (TB 17), and *Hsia-kuan* (lower passage, Stomach 7).

C) Pruritus:

According to all three of the above mentioned Chinese sources, the treatment for pruritus consists of needling *Ting-hui*, GB 2 during 8 of the patient's breaths, or else needling *Hsia-hsi,* GB 43, to a depth of 1/2 inch during seven of the patient's breaths.

D) Otalgia (Ehr-Tung):

According to the ancient Japanese this disease orginates from illnesses of the nose, tonsilitis, pharyngitis, tongue inflammation, or disease of the "pressing and joining cartilage" (*Hui-ya...*the epiglottis). According to modern concepts it is due to troubles originating in the inferior maxillary articulation, parotid or nearby lymphatics, or toothaches, The symptoms include ear inflammation, pain, difficulty in hearing and speaking.

The following are the indicated points (Diagram 20):

Acupuncture:

Hsia-kuan, St 7, 1/2 inch (*Tsun*) deep.
Ehr-men, TB 21, 6/10 inch (*Tsn*) deep.
T'ing-kung, SI 19, 1/10 inch (*Tsun*) deep.
Zu San-li, St 36, 1 inch (*Tsun*) deep.

Moxibustion:

5 moxas at SI 19 and TB 21.
7 Moxas at St 36.

For the treatment of pain localised in front of the ear, the-*Chen Chiu Yi Che* recommends the needling of *Shao-shang,* Lung 11. In the case of pain inside the ear, it is best to prick LI 11, *Ch'u-ch'ih.* (Bleeding for inflammations.)

The *Chen Chiu Ta Cheng* indicates to use *Wan-gu,* GB 12, for pain behind the ears and head-aches in general; *Zu-lin-chi'i,* GB 41, for pain at the mastoid process. If this pain should reach as far as the shoulder and elbow, then TB 10, *T'ien-ching* (Celestial Wall) should be used. For outer ear pain, or acute pain in the ear, one must disperse *Ting-hui,* GB 2 during 8 breaths. (When the mention of "breaths " is made it refers to the patient's breaths. Through a certain calculation of the flow of energy in the meridians, one can arrive at a knowledge of how many breaths are necessary to move the energy from one meridian to another.)

E) Ear inflammation, Otitis, Abcess (*Ehr-ting, Ehr-liu*): (Diagram 20)

1: External ear inflammation:
Ehr-men, TB 21.
T'ing-kung, SI 19.

2: Middle ear inflammation:
T'ing-hui, GB 2.
Wan-gu, GB 12.
Nao-hu, TM 17.

3: Inner ear inflammation:
Fung-ch'ih, GB 20.
Ch'iao-yin, GB 11.
Yi-fung, TB 17.
Chin-mai, TB 18.

4: Otitis accompanied by pus or humoral emmission:
  Hsia-kuan, St 7.
  T'ing-hui, GB 2.
  Lu-hsi, TB 19.
  Ehr-men, TB 21.

5: Otitis accompanied by temporary blockage of ears, with pain, tinnitis, chronic fever outbursts, and thickening of the tympanic membrane:
  Same points as in (4) plus:
  Yi-fung, TB 17,
  Chi-mai, TB 18,
  Wan-gu, GB 12.
  Or 7 moxas at GB 20, *Nei-kuan,* EH 6, and *Ch'ien-ku,* SI 2.

F) Tinnitis *(Ehr-ming;* Singing ears): Tinnitis is divided into three main groups in the Chinese texts, although there are numerous subdivisions. These three groups are:
  1) cicada singing (*Ch'an-ming*).
  2) big buzzing (*Hong*).
  3) little buzzing (*liao, liao chiu*).

In the *Yi Sio Jiu Men,* the following description of this disorder is given:

"Ringing in the ears may be due either to the formation of a ball of cerumen as a reaction to shock or heat, or a blocking off of energy which may eventually lead to total deafness. Some types of ringing in the ears cause excrutiating pain, giving one the impression of having insects trapped inside the ears. Others are painful because of dryness within the inner ear. In other words the origin is either shock, heat, fire, or emptiness of energy. Some are caused by insufficiency of the kidneys, or anemia.

"Most of the time, however, it is due to insufficiency of the Triple Burner, hand "minimum" *Yang* meridian, through a branch which penetrates from behind the ear, especially the superior burner."

The occidental explanation is as follows. It may be due to a prolonged usage, or abuse of quinine, antibiotics, or aspirins, or hypothyroidism. It may be a symptom of chronic nephritis, since the ringing is often on the side of the contracted and inflamed kidney. Or else, it may be due to a contraction of the hammer muscle (innervated by the inferior maxillary nerve of the trigeminal) which is pulling the tympanic membrane and pushing the stirrup into the oval foramen, causing compression and ringing. It is also often a result of cerebral anemia.

Main tympanitis points: (Diagram 20)

Ho-ku	LI 4
Kuan-Ch'ung	TB 1
Ehr-chien	LI 2
Yang-hsi	LI 5
Wan-ku	SI 4
Yieh-men	TB 2
P'ien-li	LI 6
Hsia-hsi	GB 43
Chih-yin	Bl 67
Shen-mai	Bl 62
Ehr-men	TB 21
Yi-fung	TB 17
Hsia-kuan	St 7
T'ien-liao	TB 15
Ho-liao	TB 15
Han-yan	GB 4

If the singing is due to insufficiency of the kidneys, one must needle Shen-shu (Bl 23) and Tai-hsi (Ki 3). If it is due to excessive coitus it is more recommended to use moxa, especially at Zu San-li, St 36, and at Ho-ku LI 4.

—Cicada singing in ears: The ancient and turn of the century texts indicate the following points specifically for this type of singing sound in the ears:

Zu San-li	St 36
Ti-wu-huei	GB 42
Ehr-men	TB 21
T'ing-kung	SI 19
Lieh-ch'ueh	Lu 7
Shao-chung	He 9
T'ing-hui	GB 2
Chung-ch'ung	EH 9
Shang-yang	LI 1

—**Roon Toon-toon singing (accompanied by deafness):** The name implies an alliteration as to the sound the patient hears. The points are:

    Wai-kuan . . . . TB 5
    Fu-pai. . . . . GB 10

—**Shao-shao-nong-nong:** Again, the name implies an alliteration.

    T'ing-kung . . . . SI 19
    Ho-liao . . . . TB 22

—**Pain and ringing:**

    Hou-shi. . . . . SI 3
    Pai-hui . . . . TM 20
    T'ing-hui. . . . . GB 2
    or Yi-fung, TB 17, during 7 breaths.

—**Ringing & deafness due to shock:** one must needle either Shang-yang, LI 1 or Wai-kuan, TB 5, at a depth of 1/10 inch or apply 3 moxas. If the trouble is in the left ear, one must use the points on the opposite hand, and vice-versa.

G) **Deafness:** According to the Chinese classics: "Deafness is due to a thickening of the tympanic membrane or to its perforation, or stems from birth."

The *Yi Sio Jiu Men* gives the following details: "Left and right ear are deaf when an abuse of the taste-buds (according to the theory of the five flavors) troubles the fire of the stomach." . . . Since the 5 *Yang* meridians all connect with the ears more or less directly, and the *Yin* meridians indirectly, except for the kidneys and the heart which do have direct inner channels to the ears, the emotions and chemical reactions created by an abuse of food and drink, (therefore of the taste-buds), can lead to deafness.

"The left ear is deaf when anger and bitterness troubles the fire of the gall bladder" . . Anger is the emotion associated with the liver and gall bladder. This emotion is compared to the Wind in the forest, since the liver and gall bladder correspond to the element Wood. A little wind is beneficial in spreading the seed and enlarging the boundaries of the woods, but too much wind can break the trees. In the same way, a little aggressivity (anger) is good for the liver, but too much anger can stir up the blood pressure to a dangerous level. Also certain foods and drink tend to activate the heart, and overstimulate the liver, with the possible consequence of causing deafness in the left ear. The Chinese further state that deafness, where it is not due to birth, is usually to be found on the left ear, since the majority of people suffer from repressed or over activated anger and aggressivity.

"If the right ear is deaf, then the fire of desire and licentious behaviour disturbed the fire of the conscious mind." Here again the Chinese warn us of the consequences of abuse of gratification of sex and drink, which impair the conscious mind from its normal functioning. We must find a balance of all our emotions. Even too much joy can kill as is often the case of people suffering from stroke. Here one of the results is deafness of the right ear.

Deafness can be divided in two categories, recent or old, due to insufficiency of energy or due to excessive energy.

a) **Recent:** This is due to an overabundance of fire in the hand *Yang* minimum triple burner meridian and in the foot *Yang* minimum gall bladder meridian. It may also be caused by fire (heat) in the large intestine meridian. One must get rid of the heat, shock and obstructive mucus.

b) **Chronic:** This is due to an insufficiency of the kidneys. They must be supplemented.

c) **Pulse diagnosis:** If the kidney pulse is soft and slow, this is a sign of emptiness. The kidneys must be supplemented. If the kidney pulse is superficial and quick, then the fire within the kidneys must be gotten rid off, as it can also affect the heart. If the pulse is deep and rough, this indicates that there is anger or repressed heat (aggressivity) which must be soothed.

According to the *Chen Chiu Ta Cheng*, "When the trouble lies in the secondary vessels of the large intestine meridian, there may be deafness. If one needles at LI 1 (*Shang-yang*) on both hands, the hearing will return immediately. If this doesn't help needle *Chung-ch'ung*, EH-9. For temporary deafness do not needle on the right side, as this is the side of energy, and there is a risk of aggravating the condition.

If the cause of deafness is shock, then needle the left ear for the right and the right ear for the left. In general try the large intestine meridian first, and only if this doesn't work try the triple burner of heart constrictor* meridian. . . . Sudden deafness is usually restored immediately if treated at once. The longer the illness the longer the treatment.''

The points indicated are the same as for the other ear problems, as far as local points are concerned. The only precaution is to needle opposite ears in recent or acute cases, and to try the large intestine distal points before the triple burner points, though the latter meridian is connected more closely to the ear. This is done for the simple reason that we are dealing with energy and if we needle the wrong points (especially the distal points on the extremities) we may be opening the channel for the illness to enter deeper into the organism instead of getting it out. The distal points are the ones that effect the cure. The local points merely unblock the ears but do not control them permanently.

H) The modern treatment of Deafness: According to reports from mainland China, results in treating children who are born deaf have had 80-90% success. Acupuncture is not the only technique used. Sometimes Chinese massage and physiotherapy are used in conjunction with acupuncture. Also, as soon as the slightest improvement is noticed, speech therapy is immediately applied, which has proven vital for correcting both deafness and mutism.

They have found that the longer the duration of the treatment the better the results. Therapy is continued even if results are not obtained immediately. In the Occident this is difficult to undertake, since the child's parents may not be able to afford such lengthy treatment. The treatments would almost have to be free of charge through some means, or else only wealthy parents could afford treatment for their children in this way.

The treatments are given in consecutive courses of 10 days with 3 day rest periods in between. Each time only two points are used, one local and one distal, for instance TB 21 and TB 5. The points are different every time. On the following day for instance, GB 2 and LI 4 may be used. The points used are the same as the

---

*Heart constrictor = pericardium, or envelope of the heart.

ancient points indicated in the old texts, with the exception that the needles are inserted twice as deeply as indicated in the old texts. One must be careful in needling, in that once the skin has been penetrated, no pressure should be exerted. The needle should be allowed to follow its own course, which can sometimes be quite deep. The fingers must be trained to be sensitive, since the depth is determined by the feeling of contact, twitching or electricity felt at the finger tips, which the child also feels in the ears. As soon as this sensation is felt (to be distinguished from pain), the acupuncturist may stop and either remove the needle, or move it back and forth a few times to strengthen the stimulation. In general our experience has found that the points behind the ears are more indicated for high frequency deafness than those in front of the ears. The stimulations should not be too strong otherwise the child will not return for treatment.

Acupuncturists in China have also been using several new points which are the following (Diagram 21)*:

*In the following list of points, whose location is indicated in diagram 21, the English words appearing after the Chinese name is the translation of the Chinese name of the point. The translation at times does not appear to make sense, however, this is due to the fact that some of the meanings are very difficult to understand, even for Chinese scholars.

NL means New Locus.

HN means that the loci are situated in the Head and Neck regions.

UE means Upper Extremity.

LE means Lower Extremity.

1: **T'ing-ling:** Soul of hearing . . . NL-HN-9, indicated for deafness, dumbness, tinnitis. To needle, the mouth must be opened and the needle inserted 1 1/2 inches-2 inches deep.

2: **T'ing-hsueh:** Hearing locus . . . NL-HN-8; treats deafness and dumbness. Open mouth and needle inserted perpendicularly to 1 inch-2 inches deep.

3: **T'ing-ts'ung:** Bright hearing . . . NL-HN-11; deafness and dumbness. To be needled perpendicularly to 1 1/2 inches-2 inches deep.

4: **Ting-ming:** Listening acuity . . . NL-HN-10.

5: **Hou-T'ing-huei:** Behind listening assembly . . . NL-HN-15; for tinnitis, and deafness. The needle should be slanted slightly foreward and inserted to a depth of 1 1/2 inches-2 inches.

6: **Hou-Ting-Shueh:** Behind listening locus . . . NL-HN-14; treats deafness. The needle should be inserted at a slightly slanted angle and leaning foreward, to a depth of 1/2 inch-1 inch.

7: **Hou-T'ing-kung:** Behind listening Palace . . . NL-HN-13; treats deafness. To be needled same as above point.

8: **Hou-ts'ung:** Inferior Brightness . . . NL-HN-16; needle to a depth of 3/10 inch-1/2 inch.

9: **Ch'ih-Chien:** In front of the Pond . . . NL-HN-17. Treats deafness. The needle should be slanted towards Yi-fung TB 17 and inserted to 2-2 1/2 inches.

10: **Yi-ming-hsia:** Below Shielding from Brightness . . . NL-HN-18. This point treats deafness and should be applied at an angle towards Hou-T'ing-hui, to a depth of 2 inches.

11: **Ying-hsia:** Below the Eagle . . . NL-UE-7; treats deafness and paralysis of upper limb. Needle to a depth of 1 inch-1 1/2 inches.

12: **Tsu-Yi-ts'ung:** More brightness foot point . . . NL-LE-16; treats deafness. Needle perpendicularly or slanted to a depth varying between 1 1/2 inches-3 inches.

13: **Ling-hsia:** Below the Mound (Tomb) . . . NL-LE-17. Treats deafness, gall bladder problems, including parasites. The needle should be inserted perpendicularly to a depth of 1 inch-2 inches.

DIAGRAM 20
Side of head view with meridians and points

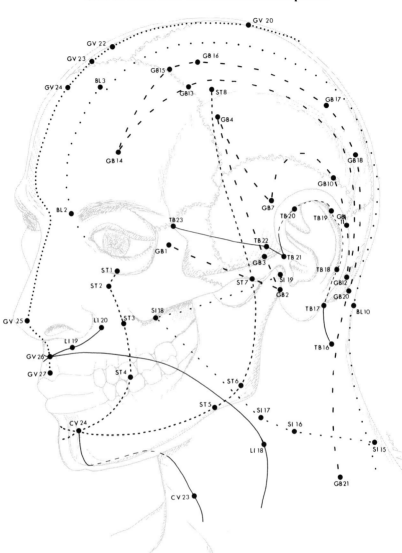

The Yang (+) meridians situated on the head and face. All of these meridians affect the sense organs either directly or indirectly through communicating branches. The main points for treating ear troubles are shown on this chart. For full effectiveness they must be combined with distal points.

DIAGRAM 21
New Ear Loci (points)

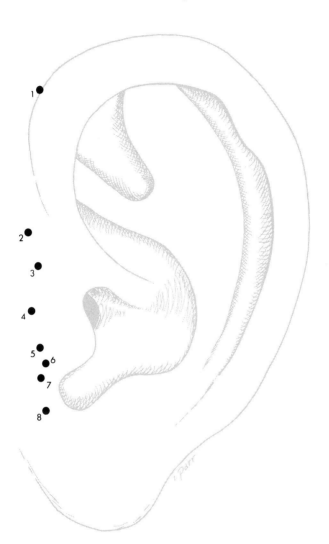

figure 1:

1. Shang-ehr-Ken (NL-HN-12)
2. Ehr-Men (TB-21)
3. CL*-HN-11
4. Ting Kung (SI-19)

5. Ting-Hsueh (NL-HN-8)
6. Ting-Ling (NL-HN-9)
7. Ting-Hui (GB-2)
8. Ting-Ming (NL-HN-10)

DIAGRAM 21
New Ear Loci (points)

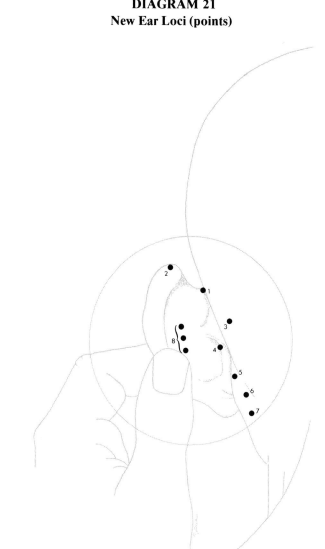

Figure 2:

1. Shang-ehr-ken (NL-HN-12)
2. CL*-HN-10
3. Hou-Ts'ung (NL-HN-16)
4. Hou-T'ing-Kung (NL-HN-13)
5. Hou-Ting-Shueh (NL-HN-14)

6. Hou-T'ing-Huei (NL-HN-15)
7. Yi-Feng (TB-17)
8. CL*-HN-12

*CL = Curious locus (ancient point
not part of meridian points)

DIAGRAM 21
New Ear Loci (points)

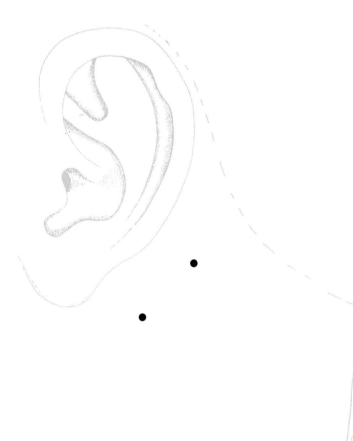

figure 3:
1. Ch'ih-Chien (NL-HN-17)
2. Yi-Ming-Hsia (NL-HN-18)

SECTION V:

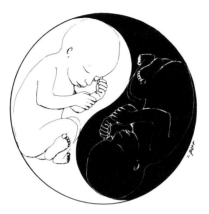

Acupuncture Anesthesia

CHAPTER 13

ACUPUNCTURE ANESTHESIA

It is no doubt the advent of acupuncture anesthesia that popularized acupuncture in America, Europe, and especially France, had been using acupuncture therapy on a large scale since 1940, which marked the creation of the International Society of Acupuncture, with its headquarters in Paris.

Acupuncture anesthesia was officially introduced to modern hospitals in China in 1958 and is the result of a chance discovery made by Chinese acupuncturists. It began with the treatment of postoperative sore throat, the inability to eat and drink, which are usual complications following tonsillectomy under local anesthesia.

Acupuncture was known to be highly effective in the treatment of pharyngitis and other throat ailments. Thus the postoperative complaints were treated easily by acupuncture.

Eventually the question arose as to why acupuncture could not also prevent this condition, since the Chinese classics maintained that acupuncture was above all a preventive form of medicine. This was done and the results were successful. Therefore the first operation done under acupuncture anesthesia was a tonsillectomy. Even today almost all tonsillectomies in China are performed in this way.

At the same time it was discovered the acupuncture could be used to prevent pain during the cleansing of wounds and little by little it was experimented in every type of surgery. One of its obvious advantages was the reduction of narcotics by 80%.

Mechanism of Action:

Although acupuncture anesthesia has proven its efficiency around the world its mechanism of action has not yet been discovered. Naturally we can only try to explain it through the neurophysiological notions of pain that we possess, which are still fragmentary.

Our senses are a means of communicating, that our organism has at its disposal. Pain is an entirely different mechanism, however, and does not constitute a normal physiological state. There is no sense of pain as there is a sense of touch or sight. On the contrary pain is the result of an imbalance or disruption of the normal physiological state of the body. It is a pathological condition which serves to warn the subject of imminent danger in order to stimulate the defenses towards recovery and protection. Although it can be beneficial if it is only a brief sensation, it is highly dangerous when prolonged over a period of time and leads to a complete disruption of the normal mental and physiological organisation of the individual.

The action of pain on the whole being, emotional, intellectual and physical, makes it all the more difficult to analyse and measure its mechanism, since it implies an interaction of the entire nervous structure. Adding to this factors such as individual variability, variety of types of expression, lack of specific stimuli, and its predominent personal aspect we are all the more at an impass to interpret it scientifically.

Many experiments have been carried out in such an endeavor; however, every theory that has been developed has eventually fallen before the inscrutability of scientific analysis and we remain at an impass. Histology, for instance, does not possess the instruments necessary to follow the paleo-spino-reticulo-thalamic pathway which forms a vast and diffused network, intermingling with many anatomical structures and leading to a variety of subcortical and cortical structures. It cannot detect all the interconnections and targets of pain which are spread out at the different levels of the nervous system and mostly at the higher centers.

We might conclude however, that though we do not understand the physiology of pain entirely, enough is understood to entertain the hope of a possible solution in the near future. Although a scientific explanation to the mechanism of acupuncture analgesia is a highly complicated matter, its practical application is simple.

Induction Time:

In general an induction time of 20-30 minutes is necessary to produce an anesthetic effect strong enough to permit surgery. Once this state is reached the operation can begin and the patient remains conscious at all times. His senses are in tact at all times. The only sense which is diminished is the receptivity to pain. Acupuncture anesthesia seems to have a hypoanalgesic effect on pain in the desired area of the body, since the sense of touch does not diminish. The patient can still feel the blade cutting through the skin, though there is no pain sensation.

In the beginning there seems to be a rise in blood pressure, blood sugar, adrenaline output and pulse. This seems to be due to stress caused by the atmosphere of the operating room. These quickly return to normal, and only then is it possible to commence operating. To observe the proper induction time is of course as important as choosing the right points.

Selection of points:

In the beginning as many as one hundred needles were used in certain operations and it was necessary to have as many as four or five acupuncturists in the operating room twirling the needles manually for a considerable length of time. This represented many inconveniences: the fatigue on the part of the acupuncturist who had to exert a tremendous effort in stimulating the needles manually, while paying constant attention to every fluctuation of the patient's state and working in harmony with the other acupuncturists, the reduced space alloted to the surgeon, and the dramatic effect so many people attending to him must have had on the patient.

The number of points was eventually reduced, which did not lessen the anesthetic effect but on the contrary, augmented it. Today many operations require only one needle. However, it is found by using only one local needle and one distal needle a greater electromagnetic field, or loop, seems to be developed. Also, the stimulation need no longer be manual, since electrical stimulation can be used to facilitate the task.

It seems that the points which are most useful during operations are those which produce a greater sensation of "Teh Chi" or "take" as it is sometimes translated. This sensation can be described as producing a feeling of heaviness, numbness, tingling, cold or heat which can spread out along an entire limb or part of the body. The acupuncturist knows when this sensation is being felt by the patient because he feels as though the needle were suddenly being gripped by some force of a magnetic nature. This sensation must be differentiated from pain.

Thus the amount of needles was diminished at the same time as the amount of points found to be useful. These were brought down to 29; only those that produced greater sensations of "take" or "teh chi" were used. Specific points have also been found to act on specific parts of the body. In other words, what the ancient Chinese said thousands of years ago has been found not only to be true, but can in fact be used in modern laboratories.

The Ear:

Since 1969, thousands of operations have been carried out in China using the ear points, for every type of surgery.

Since the nerves covering the ear are derived from larger nerves originating in different areas of the body, the ear points can be used to stimulate, and therefore also to anesthetize, every part of the body. (See Diagram 3)

How this came about was by the discovery that during gastrectomy, the stomach point on the ear became sensitive to touch and that this eventually spread out to other surrounding points. Thus by needling this point an analgesic effect was obtained. Similar findings in other operations have encouraged the use of ear points in anesthesia. Dr. Roccia of Italy, who has certainly done more operations under acupuncture anesthesia than any other occidental (500 to date) uses the ear points in almost every operation.

A few examples of acupuncture anesthesia using the ear points

TONSILLECTOMY

Ear points:

> Larynx and Pharynx
> Tonsil

After the age of 5 years, a third needle is placed on the helix. An additional needle is added on the helix for every 10 years of age. They are placed on the right ear to facilitate the task of the surgeon and must not be twirled or stimulated. For full efficiency, the needles should be inserted rapidly and firmly despite the movements of the child.

Body points: Ho-ku LI 4, is placed bilaterally. Only the needle on the right hand should be twisted or stimulated during the entire operation. The left one is merely left standing.

Induction time: 5-6 minutes.

Remarks: Children, remarkable as it may seem, usually remain calm during the entire procedure. The analgesic effect remains after the operation, which can be easily seen by the fact that the child can eat almost right away.

The gag reflex can be eliminated by having the patient practice with a tongue depressor in his throat the day prior to the operation.

Dental Extractions

The points are selected according to the area to be operated.

Ear points:

> Tooth extraction point-1 (upper jaw)
> Tooth extraction point-2 (lower jaw)
> Toothache point (the needle must be directed toward the diseased tooth).

The ear points are done on the side to be operated.

Body Points: The needle is inserted at a 30-45 degree angle from Sanchien, LI 3, through to Ho-ku LI 4. It must be manipulated during the entire operation.

Electrical stimulation: The corresponding tooth extraction point and the toothache point on the ear are stimulated together, first for 1-2 minutes, allowing a five minute rest, then again for another 1-2 minutes. Thus a total induction time of 7-10 minutes is necessary preceding the operation. After surgery the ear needles are removed first and the needle at LI 4 allowed to remain in place for a further 5 minutes to ensure analgesia.

Analgesic blockage: From 1970-72, the Tai Yuan no. 4 hospital conducted a series of experiments using analgesic blockage of auricular points with 0.3-1 ml. of physiological serum injected into the points. This produced 10 minutes later a sensation of numbness, tension and heat, which corresponded to the induction time after which surgery was possible.

97.1% success was obtained with 1250 tooth extractions of this type, with 65.6% very good results. The most effective points were found to be the tooth extraction points 1 & 2.

PULMONARY SURGERY

Ear points:
corresponding Lung
External Nose

These points are connected and stimulated electrically.

Body points: Nei-kuan (EH 6) is used to a depth of 0.5-1.5 inches. Pi Yong, LI 14, is also used quite often. Any one of the above two points can be used alone without any other point, which seems quite unbelievable for such a complex operation.

Precautions: In order to avoid mediastinal flutter during paradoxal respiration and substernal pressure during the operation, the patient is taught abdominal breathing as soon as he is hopsitalized. He is instructed about everything that he might feel when the chest is open and how to breathe at such a time to avoid complications and oppression. The best results were obtained with patients who could breathe 6-8 times in one minute, during one half hour.

Intercostal nerve block with 1% procaine is frequently practiced to prevent pain from the skin incision and rib resection. Sometimes a local anesthetic is used such as 0.25% procaine (10-30 ml) and 50-150 mg of Dolantin intravenously, may also be prescribed.

The surgeon must avoid touching the lungs or diaphragm with his fingers. When the bronchi are being manipulated, the patient is instructed to breathe deeply with his mouth open to prevent the cough reflex. Sometimes a peribronchial infiltration of procaine is necessary.

Because the analgesic effect is usually not complete the operation must be done as quickly as possible, the skin must be sutured immediately.

For patients with large amounts of expectoration and very poor pulmonary functions, endotracheal intubation is recommended. A preliminary spray of anesthetic in the throat is often necessary for intubation.

SPLENECTOMY

305 cases of late schistosomiasis were operated in Changshan County People's Hospital with a success rate of 95.5%. The best results were obtained by combining ear points with nose points. The ear points are deemed to provide a strong inhibitory effect on the traction sensation while the nose points provide analgesia and muscle relaxation, which is a most important factor in this type of operation.

Ear points:
Sympathetic
Shen Men
Lung
Spleen

DIAGRAM 22
Nose Therapy points

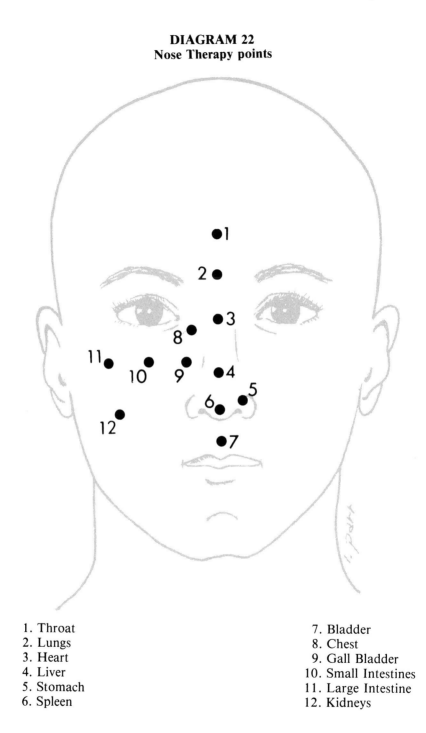

1. Throat
2. Lungs
3. Heart
4. Liver
5. Stomach
6. Spleen

7. Bladder
8. Chest
9. Gall Bladder
10. Small Intestines
11. Large Intestine
12. Kidneys

Nose points: The most effective points were the Lung and Spleen points. (see Diagram 22). The needle must pass subcutaneously from the Lung point through to the Spleen point. This direction is most important.

Stimulation:

The intensity and frequency vary with each individual. The optimal frequency varies from 150-200 cycles per minute with an intensity of 4-7 mA. These also vary with age and sex, being higher in males than females and higher in adolescents than in children and elderly people.

The induction time is usually about 30-40 minutes, but can last longer.

Pre-operative Preparation:

The patient must be prepared psychologically and told exactly what he may feel and what will be done throughout the operation.

The day prior to the operation he is given very light meals, mostly liquid, and no enema or gastric decompression is necessary.

One hour before the operation 0.1-0.2 gm of sodium luminal are injected intramuscularly or 0.2-0.6 gm of meprobamate are prescribed.

Per-operative adjuvants:

During the operation, 50 mg of Dolantin and 25 mg of promethazine hydrochloride (phenergan) by slow intravenous dripping are administered. The dose must be reduced, to prevent sleepiness, which would hinder cooperation between surgeon and patient.

10-30 ml of 0.5% procaine are injected into the muscular layer after the skin incision.

This form of operation has the added benefit of reducing the required hospitalization time from 35 to 25 days.

EVALUATING ACUPUNCTURE ANESTHESIA

Since its inception in 1958, over 400,000 operations have been performed in China under acupuncture anesthesia, for every type of surgery, minor and major. A success rate of 90% was obtained over all, with 60-65% good or very good results. The advantages of this method are numerous:

. . . It is a simple and highly economical procedure, requiring only a few needles and an electrical stimulator which can be built for a few dollars.

. . . The life-insurance risk is non-existent, whereas the risk with general anesthesia is extremely high. The latter is considered to be the cause of one in three thousand deaths during operations.

. . . There is no drastic effect on blood pressure, whereas with general anesthesia the drastic cardiovascular perturbations are one of the major concerns of anesthetists. Hypodynamia cordis and vascular collapse resulting from operative shock are non-existent. Arterial tension and pulse rate remain relatively stable.

. . There is no drastic effect on respiration and practically no apnea as in general anesthesia.

. . . There is practically no digestive risk and therefore it is not necessary to have an empty stomach to undergo surgery. This presents an obvious advantage in the case of emergencies.

. . . There is no interference in renal and hepatic functions.

. . . Hemostasis is increased, thus erasing the risk of hemorraging.

. . . The patient need not be surveyed in the post-operative phase, as he is awake throughout the operation. He can often walk on the very same day.

. . . It prevents post-operative shock, which remains one of the major problems in general anesthesia. Other problems which are commonly encountered such as headache, vomitting, retention of urine, constipation and dyspepsia are eliminated.

. . . The analgesic effect persists throughout the post-operative phase, which precludes the necessity to administer other analgesics.

. . . The risk of infection is nonexistent. This is due to the fact that the patient remains conscious at all times and therefore does not lower his resistence.

. . . It permits a cooperation between the patient and the surgeon which isn't possible under general anesthesia and which is one of the main factors determining the failure of certain types of operations. Statistics from China show that success rates of only 4% under general anesthesia for certain types of operations, were raised to 70% under acupuncture anesthesia. For instance in a strabismus operation, the patient can cooperate with the surgeon and every movement can be appreciated with precision. In neurosurgery, it allows for early detection of hematoma and postoperative cerebral abcess which can lead to mental problems. In thyroidectomy, loss of voice by cutting the recurrent laryngeal nerve can be avoided as the patient can be asked to speak. In operations to repair tendons and muscles, the patient can remain mobile at all times, enabling the surgeon to test the results of the operation immediately.

. . . It can be used in weak and frail people who are in no condition to undergo general anesthesia.

Nevertheless, acupuncture anesthesia does present certain drawbacks:

. . . Pain is not entirely eliminated. It varies with the anatomical layers. In general the muscular fascia respond better than the deeper or more superficial layers. Local anesthsia is often necessary before cutaneous incision.

. . . It does not always protect the patient from neuro-vegetative reactions (vomitting, nausea) due to traction on the internal organs. Neither does it offer protection from external ventilatory problems such as oppression or dyspnea, associated with opening the thorax.

. . . Muscle relaxants are often necessary in abdominal surgery and in O.R.L.

. . . It does not diminish consciousness, which makes it necessary to carefully choose the type of patient to undergo this type of surgery. Hyperemotional, hypersensitive, neurotic or psychopathic individuals are necessarily excluded.

When one weighs the advantages against the disadvantages, one must admit that acupuncture anesthesia is one of the greatest achievements of modern anesthesiology. It is still in the experimental stage, being no more than some 17 years old and thus still a minor. Nevertheless it has every possibility of maturing prosperously with time, in the good hands of the modern scientist. We must not forget that western anesthesiology was once a child, and not too long ago at that.

AFTERWORD

In the preceding pages, the basic principles of ear acupuncture have been set forth. These included concepts of diagnosis through the auricle. It must be made clear, however, that auricle diagnosis does not supplant traditional scientific examination. In cases where medical examinations are useless, or are in disagreement, which is more often the case, the ear method can help to give a clearer picture of the real cause and type of disease. Moreover, in emergency cases, where there is no time to await the results of lab tests, ear examination and treatment may often save someone's life.

To date, man has not yet discovered the "fountain of youth, or bliss" in any form of therapy. Ear acupuncture is not a panacea, but it is certainly a wonderful and reliable adjunct in the hands of any competent therapist.

To quote a phrase from Shakespeare's Hamlet, which I think is most applicable today, in our rapidly changing society,....

"There are more things in heaven and earth, Horatio, than are dreamt of in your philosophy."

BIBLIOGRAPHY

Amber, R.B. and Babey-Brooke, A.M. *The Pulse in Occident and Orient.* Dunshaw Press, New York 1966.

American Journal of Chinese Medicine (Vol. 2, No. 2, April 1974) Frederick F. Kao, Garden City, N.Y.

An Explanatory Book of the Newest Illustrations of Acupuncture Points, Medicine & Health Publishing Co., Hong Kong, July 1973.

Berlewi, Miriam, *Dictionnaire des Symboles* 1973, Ed. Seghers & Ed. Jupiter, Paris.

Drugs & Society, Vol. 2, #8, May 1973. MacMillian Journals, London.

Ear Illustration showing Acupuncture Points, East Wind Medical Instruments Co., Ltd. Hong Kong.

Lowe, William, *Introduction to Acupuncture Anesthesia*, Hans Huber Publishers, Bern, Stuttgart, Vienna. 1973.

Nanking army ear acupuncture team, *Ear Acupuncture,* Rodale Press, Inc. Book Division, Emmaus, Penn. 18049, 1974.

Nogier, P.F.M., *Traité d'Auriculothérapie,* Maisonneuve, 1969. Paris, France (also in English as *Treatise of Auriculotherapy,* 1972)

Santaro, M., *L'Acupuncture par l'Oreille,* Maloine, Paris, 1974.

Soulié de Morant, George, *L'Acupuncture Chinoise,* Maloine S.A. Ed., Paris 1972.

Van Nghi, Nguyen, *Théorie et pratique de l'Analgésie par l'Acupuncture*, SOCEDIM, 1974. Marseille, France.

APPENDIX I

Therapuncteur:
MED-E-PRISE
1335 West Washington St.
Orlando, Flor. 32805   phone: (305) 843-7530

Pellin's Stigmascope:
20, Boulevard Joseph-Vallier, 38 - Grenoble, France

Acuprobe 11, model AP11:
Doctor's Supply, 24028 Union, Michigan 48124
phone: (313) 278-2840
             or
Intertronic Systems Ltd., 980 Alness St., #15,
Downsview, Ontario, Canada M3J 2S2   phone: (416) 661-3902

Auricuprobe-1:
International Acupuncture Products, Ltd.
P.O. Box 3212, Darien, Conn. 06820   phone: (203) 655-0800

Pro-Med 1100:
Professional Medical Distributors, Inc.
29830 Beck Road, Wixom, Mich. 48096   phone: (313) 624-6413

DIAGRAM 23
Indian Ear Acupuncture points

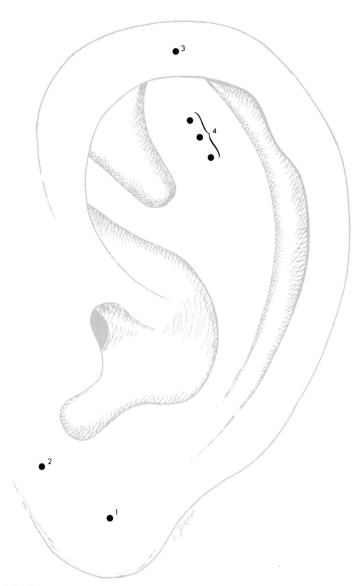

1. Vitality
2. Bronchial asthma
3. Allergy, Dermatology, Appendicitis
4. Piles

APPENDIX II

EAR ACUPUNCTURE IN INDIA
Abstract from an interview with Dr. Chandrashekhar Thakkur

I have shown in the first part of this book that many countries possessed acupuncture in one form or another. However, no detailed mention was made of India, which has had acupuncture for the past 7000 years. Whether it arrived there from China or vice-versa is difficult to ascertain. There are exponents of both theories.

If we go back to the Indian medical classics, known as the Vedas, said to be written about 7000 years ago, we find "needle therapy" mentioned there. This actually antedates the Chinese classical medical books by several millenia. One volume of the Vedas, known as the *Suchi Veda*, translated as the "art of piercing with a needle", was written about 3000 years ago and deals entirely with acupuncture.

The Indians have both body acupuncture and ear acupuncture. In the former, they have 180 points* situated in different parts of the body, which they either burn with an herb, massage or pierce with various types of needles. The methods are essentially the same as those used by the Chinese, even though the Indians have only one half the amount of points the Chinese do. Both philosophies resemble one another in that they treat Man as a microcosm, possessing in his body the same basic principles as those present in the Cosmos. Thus as with the Chinese, certain parts of the body are said to be "ruled" by Venus, others by Jupiter, and so on. All this really means, on a practical level, is that certain definite qualities are ascribed to the planets, in an effort to place the Cosmos in the functions and organs of the human body, to interrelate the two.

---

*Known as Marma: said to heal or kill.

Just as the Chinese described the basic elements in existence as five basic types, earth, metal, water, wood (sap), fire, and their composites, the Indians described four basic types. To quote Dr. Jean Schatz of Paris "It is these basic elements, in both medical philosophies, and the set rules which govern their interplay which make of these ancient forms of medicine a science."

The doctrine formed by the rules governing the interaction between the elements, is useful on many levels, one of the most important of these being the classification of the patient as belonging essentially to one type more than another. In other words, a patient belonging to the fire temperament or element would not be treated in the same way as one belonging to a water temperament. Patients can also be composites of several elements, which make up their personality. The existence of this type of doctrine greatly facilitates the task of treating the patient, by merely finding out which element is out of harmony with the others.

One will not argue the fact that acupuncture was more developed by the Chinese than the Indians and presented to us in a more scientific and complete fashion. However, the Indians have been using ear acupuncture longer than the Chinese. Let us not forget that ear acupuncture is a fairly recent development (1956) in Mainland China. It has always existed, but 90% of the points are no more than a quarter of a century old.

When a child is born in India, it is the custom to have a horoscope cast to see the most auspicious moments in his life to make certain changes for his progress and health. A date is also charted for him or her to have the ears pierced. Regardless of sex, the ears are pierced in children, not for an ornamental purpose, but to stimulate vitality (diagram 23) and to provide immunity against disease. Experience has also shown that the ear piercing helps a child in his teething, by eliminating the usual feverish condition and diarrhea.

Ayurveda or the "Science of Life" is the traditional form of medicine which is India's heritage from the past few millenia. Traditionally, the ears are described in the Ayurvedic classics as being a type of lotus, or outer flowering of the internal organs, and particularly of the kidneys, which they greatly resemble in shape. Thus kidney disorders were originally the main diseases which were diagnosed by the ears. There is a definite relationship with the Chinese here, who ascribe the same symbolism and characteristics to the ears. Eventually, the ears were taken separately and were regarded as a microcosm of their own, which reflected everything going on in the larger universe, which was the entire body. Thus, in India, an entire system of treating every type of disease by the ear alone was developed.

For instance, in treating bronchial asthma, a certain point on the lobule of the ear is pierced. The results are apparently remarkable. A point on top of the helix of the ear, which strangely enough corresponds to Dr. Nogier's allergy point, is used to treat allergy, dermatoligical disorders, to cure or prevent appendicitis.

A point on the antehelix of the auricle treats piles.

According to whether it is a male or a female patient we must use either the right or the left ear. For a female we would use the left ear and for a male the right. Curiously in China it is said to be just the opposite: left for a male and right for a female. However, many Chinese texts have been badly translated because of the similarity of ideographs which have opposite or quite different meanings.

From my point of view, certain aspects of Indian acupuncture must be taken into consideration, as they may serve to shed light on the mystery of some of the Chinese texts which have been misinterpreted. For instance the term for Pulse in Chinese* is almost written exactly the same way as the term for Mou, or energetic pathway. This means that when the Chinese text speaks of taking the pulse it may actually mean measuring the energy flow along the meridians, which has a completely different connotation. Many Chinese texts are not understood even by the Chinese, unless they are at the same time experts in medicine and experts in literature. Since the Chinese philosophies have much in common with the Indian philosophy, one may serve to clarify the other. India's medical heritage is certainly as great as China's. We must not forget that if it weren't for the Chinese revolution, acupuncture wouldn't be where it is today. It was jealously guarded by each family as its own secret and when that family died there was a good chance that its medical secrets were forgotten as well. The revolution obliged each person, though by force, to share his information with everyone else. In India today, if every family shared its medical secrets as the Chinese have, we would probably find methods quite as interesting and as effective as the Chinese ones.

LIST OF ABBREVIATIONS

He . . . . Heart meridian

SI . . . . Small Intestine meridian

Bl . . . . Bladder meridian

Ki . . . . Kidney meridian

EH or Pc. . . . . Envelope of the heart meridian, known also as the Heart Constrictor or Pericardium meridian

TB or SC. . . . . Triple Burner meridian or San Chiao (Jiao) meridian.

GB. . . . . Gall Bladder meridian

Li . . . . Liver meridian

Lu . . . . Lung meridian

LI . . . . Large Intestine meridian

St. . . . . Stomach meridian

Sp . . . . Spleen (& Pancreas) meridian

TM or Gv . . . . Tu Mo, the Governing vessel

JM, or RM, or CV . . . . Jen Mo, also written Ren Mo, the Conception vessel

Dr. Mario Wexu first became acquainted with the art of acupuncture at the age of three, when he received his first treatment from his father, Dr. Oscar Wexu, a skilled acupuncturist. He studied Physical Education, Philosophy, Sociology, Physiotherapy and Osteopathy. He gained first hand knowledge of different societies and their healing techniques while traveling through Europe, North Africa, Asia and North America.

His father taught him acupuncture and later sent him to perfect his skill in Hong Kong, under the apprenticeship of an old friend, Dr. Lok Yee-Kung (President of the Hong Kong College of Chinese Medicine and Acupuncture), now in Las Vegas, and to learn the famous "pulse diagnosis" technique under the late Dr. King-Ying. Upon returning to Montreal in 1971, he helped his father establish the first legal Association of Acupuncture in North America. Dr. Wexu practices acupuncture, lectures and teaches at the Quebec Institute of Acupuncture, where he is presently Director of Studies.

He is a graduate of the China Applied Acupuncture College of Hong Kong and the Hong Kong College of Chinese Medicine and Acupuncture. He is Vice-President of the Quebec Association of Acupuncture; Director of the Montreal Center of Chinese Massotherapy; Council Member of the World Academic Society of Acupuncture, and is a member of the International Society of Acupuncture.

ACUPUNCTURE AND THE LIFE ENERGIES

The author, Dr. Sidney Rose-Neil, has been interested in and involved with Nature Cure and Acupuncture for many years. He sees Acupuncture as a natural part of his holistic approach to health. While diet, correct posture, breathing and exercise all play a part in health, there are also imbalances produced which require adjustment rather than dramatic change.

Acupuncture provides just such a dimension, an opening of channels to release the flow of vital energy, the body's own healing forces. This in turn led Dr. Rose-Neil to develop his thinking along the lines expressed in this book.

This book provides a non-material explanation consistent with the many inexplicable phenomena posed by healing through the ages. It starts from the premise that "There is no such thing as a miracle, only unknown laws" and leads by a variety of paths to the inevitable conclusion that it is *energy* which provides the underlying blue-print.

ACUPUNCTURE AND THE LIFE ENERGIES investigates these vital energies through a wide variety of different topics. Among these are: *The Kirilian Effect, Magnets and Magnetic Healing, Biofeedback, Orgone Therapy, Electro-Acupuncture, Bodily Clocks, Cycles* and more.

**ASI Publishers Inc., 127 Madison Avenue
New York, N.Y. 10016**

Cover design by Melissa Zorn

ISBN 0-88231-121-2

ACUPUNCTURE THERAPY
Dr. Mary Austin

This is the comprehensive textbook of Chinese acupuncture in the English language.

The author, who practices acupuncture and osteopathy, describes in a clear and straightforward manner the complete range of acupuncture techniques, with anatomical references to the structure of the human body.

Dr. Austin presents through text and many detailed illustrations the precise locations of all acupuncture points along the 12 organ meridians (or pathways of energy), as well as the points on the two major vessel meridians. When manipulated by needle, massage, perscussion, or Moxa, these points can help **balance deficiencies and** excesses within the body.

The Yin-Yang symbol represents the bi-polar energy permeating every cell and tissue of living organisms. Acupuncture is the art of balancing these negative (Yin) and these positive (Yang) forces by the manipulation of points along the energy pathways of the body.

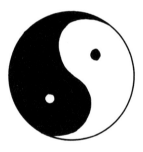

The text is well suited for doctors, nurses, students, and others seriously interested in understanding this art and science of healing.

ISBN: 0-88231-003-8

INTRODUCTION TO AYURVEDA

By Dr. Chandrashekhar G. Thakkur

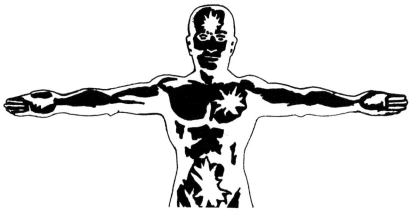

What is Ayurveda? Literally, it means "the Science of Life." (Ayur = Life, Veda = Science.) But this traditional Indian system of medicine covers not only the knowledge of life, but the knowledge of healthy living as well.

As with Acupuncture, the Ayurvedic principles are as useful today as when they were first expounded thousands of years ago; yet they remain largely unknown in the Western world. It is hoped the publication of INTRODUCTION TO AYURVEDA will help correct this unfortunate omission.

A PARTIAL LISTING OF CONTENTS INCLUDES:

* The Five Element Theory.
* Anatomy in Ayurveda.
* The Tridosha Theory of Vayu, Pitta and Kapha, which in normal balance sustain health, while their imbalance causes the physical unhappiness known as "Roga" or disease.
* Examination of a patient and principles of treatment.
* Art and Science of Pharmacy.

ISBN: 0-88231-005-4

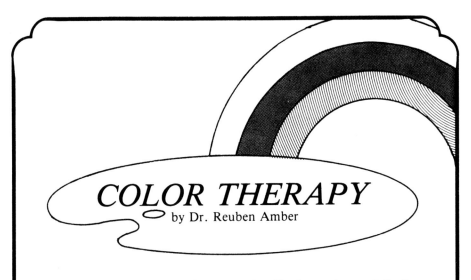

COLOR THERAPY
by Dr. Reuben Amber

Color is a vibration that is constantly affecting us in our daily lives. This book enumerates the myriad ways we can choose to consciously use color to influence our body, mind and soul to promote balanced health and well being.

Part I on the theory and philosophy of Chromotherapy begins with an historical survey of mythology from different parts of the world, drawing heavily on ancient Ayurvedic (Hindu medical) lore. The views of modern light physics, radionics as well as the work of well known researchers including Burr, De La Warr, Reich and Steiner are then presented.

Part II gives specific applications of color in our environment, with our food, clothing and light, sensitizing us to the healing power or the destructive effects of a guided use of color therapy. This section on the practice of Chromotherapy includes: how to heal with color, auras, the individual healing properties of each color and their use for specific diseases. Dr. Amber also provides valuable techniques for color treatment in relation to solarized water, visualizations gems, color breathing, chakra therapy and planetary correspondences. A unique feature is the inclusion of an extensive repertory listing the relationship of color, tast, polarity, organs, elements and diseases, to foster a holistic use of these techniques.

This book is valuable and important not only for healing already existing physical imbalances, but ideally to help us become more aware of how color can create a positive balance within ourselves and our environment.

ISBN 0-88231-067-4

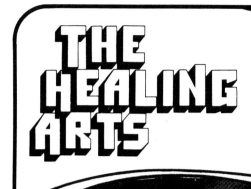

HOW ATMOSPHERIC CONDITIONS AFFECT YOUR HEALTH

By Dr. Michel Gauquelin

Deaths are more frequent when a weather front passes over. Fogs kill, winds devastate, sudden drops in barometric pressure and electrical agitation in the air affect man—why? and how?

In answering these questions Dr. Gauquelin also postulates the fascinating question of the effect of cosmic influences on our health. Formerly they were not separated from atmospheric conditions. Now, new scientific research reveals the legitimate relationship between the two.

First published in 1971, this new second edition updates the discoveries that have been made since then, about the weather and our health.

Dr. Michel Gauquelin is a Sorbonne trained psychologist and statistician. Since 1969, he has been the director of the *Laboratory for the Study of the Relationship between Cosmic and Psycho-Physicological Rhythms* in Paris, France. An accomplished writer, he is the author of numerous works in the fields of psychology and cosmic science.

ISBN:0-88231-066-6

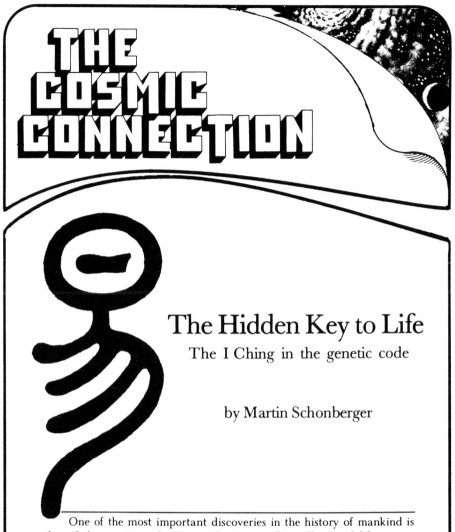

THE COSMIC CONNECTION

The Hidden Key to Life
The I Ching in the genetic code

by Martin Schonberger

One of the most important discoveries in the history of mankind is that of the genetic code. Every planet as well as all animal life is now recognized as having come into existence, being formed and multiplied by *64 code words* written on the long-chain molecule DNA.

The universal claims of both the I-Ching, "the book of changes," the compendium of Chinese natural knowledge, and the genetic code, "the book of life," encouraged the author to establish the hypothesis of a *general system* in nature. He has verified in numerous parallels the congruence of both the I-Ching code and the genetic code. These sensational results are detailed for the first time in this book.

ISBN 0-88231-023-2

(G)

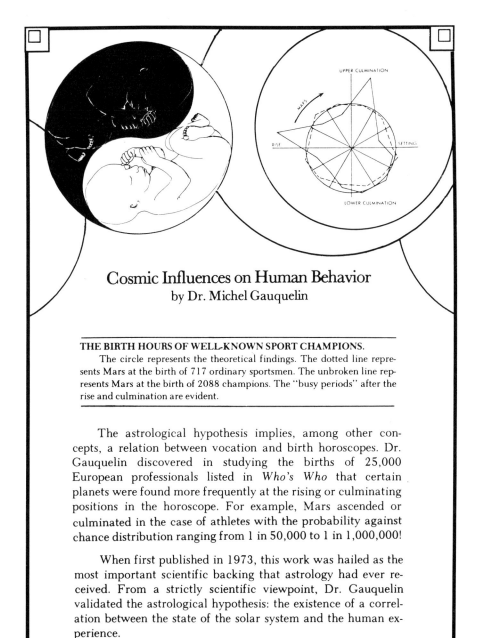

Cosmic Influences on Human Behavior
by Dr. Michel Gauquelin

THE BIRTH HOURS OF WELL-KNOWN SPORT CHAMPIONS.
The circle represents the theoretical findings. The dotted line represents Mars at the birth of 717 ordinary sportsmen. The unbroken line represents Mars at the birth of 2088 champions. The "busy periods" after the rise and culmination are evident.

The astrological hypothesis implies, among other concepts, a relation between vocation and birth horoscopes. Dr. Gauquelin discovered in studying the births of 25,000 European professionals listed in *Who's Who* that certain planets were found more frequently at the rising or culminating positions in the horoscope. For example, Mars ascended or culminated in the case of athletes with the probability against chance distribution ranging from 1 in 50,000 to 1 in 1,000,000!

When first published in 1973, this work was hailed as the most important scientific backing that astrology had ever received. From a strictly scientific viewpoint, Dr. Gauquelin validated the astrological hypothesis: the existence of a correlation between the state of the solar system and the human experience.

This new second edition updates Dr. Gauquelin's research and includes his latest findings on the planetary factors in personality.